Practice Check!

The Professional Developments Series

These five books have been developed from articles previously published in *The Professional Nurse* magazine to provide you with a wealth of insight into all aspects of nursing practice. The series is essential reading for qualified nurses who need to keep up with new developments, evaluate their clinical practice and develop and extend their clinical, management and teaching skills. Up-to-date, and appropriately illustrated, The Professional Developments Series brings together the work of over a hundred authors and will be of wide interest to nurses in every health care setting.

Other titles in The Professional Developments Series:

The Ward Sister's Survival Guide

This book is essential reading and valuable reference for all nurses with direct clinical management responsibility.

Patient Education Plus

This book will help you to develop your teaching role with patients and clients, and covers a wide range of clinical topics. Each chapter includes a clearly written and illustrated handout which can be freely photocopied or adapted for use with your clients.

The Staff Nurse's Survival Guide

Relevant to nurses working in all healthcare settings, this brings together chapters on a wide range of clinical and non-clinical issues in patient care, and includes a practical section on looking after *yourself*, too.

Effective Communication

Good communication is an essential part of effective nursing, and this title in the series covers a wide range of topics, including counselling, confidentiality, group and team work, compliance and communicating with children.

These books are available from the publishers:

Austen Cornish Publishers Limited
Brook House
2–16 Torrington Place
London WC1E 7LT
Tel: 071-636 4622

Ask to be included on their mailing list!

Practice Check!

A collection of Practice Check articles
first published in The Professional Nurse
and here revised and updated

Austen Cornish Publishers Limited
London
1990

Practice Check!
First published in 1990. Reprinted 1990

Austen Cornish Publishers Limited
Brook House
2–16 Torrington Place
London WC1E 7LT

© Austen Cornish Publishers Limited 1990

ISBN 1 870065 10 7

Printed and bound in Great Britain by Richard Clay Limited,
Bungay, Suffolk.

Contents

How to use Practice Check!

These Practice Checks were first published as articles in *The Professional Nurse* magazine. They have been updated and brought together in this single volume.

There are many situations which arise in nursing practice in which there are no clear 'right answers'. Nurses need to decide (often quickly) how best to handle these. Practice Checks are designed to enable you to explore some of these situations by presenting brief descriptions of the problems which can arise, and then asking you open-ended questions about them. The authors have provided some thoughts and ideas about the best options in these situations but they leave plenty of scope for you to think through the issues which arise whenever effective communication between people is required. Communicating with elderly people, children, anxious people and those who are dying are all addressed in different Practice Checks. Attitudes towards Aids victims and people who are mentally ill are challenged, and thought-provoking situations requiring the development of partnership with patients are also presented. Three Practice Checks cover clinical subject matter and give you a chance to test your knowledge and practice.

When these articles were first published in the magazine, they were widely welcomed by readers, many of whom collected them for future use. Ward sisters, community nurses and tutors found them particularly valuable as a focus for group discussion with colleagues and students about a particular problem area. You can easily add more examples from the situations which arise with your own patients and colleagues! Other readers found them a valuable and thought-provoking way of challenging their own understanding of a difficult or unclear aspect of their own practice.

Because of their potential value to groups of nurses, the publishers are taking the unusual step of freeing the normal copyright restrictions which usually prevent readers from photocopying material from books and magazines. *For educational use only* and *not* for re-sale in any form, these Practice Checks can be photocopied without permission in writing from the publisher.

Elizabeth M Horne
Editorial Director, The Professional Nurse,
London, September 1989

Practice Check!

There is a myth in nursing that communicating with elderly people follows a routine pattern, needing only basic skills, when in fact unskilled communication can have devastating effects on the lives of elderly people. To what extent is your practice based on sound principles?

Communicating with elderly people

Kevin Teasdale, MA, Cert Ed, RMN
Director of In-Service Training and Post Basic Nurse Education, Pilgrim Hospital, Boston, Lincs.

Personal relationships can be seen as a series of bargains, negotiated from differing positions of power. This Exchange Theory suggests that as people enter the later stages of their lives, they have less to bargain with – physically, materially and socially. They are then vulnerable to learned helplessness – the belief that whatever actions they take, they can no longer get what they want, no longer control their environment or the ways in which they organise their life – resulting in a state of apathy, passiveness and introversion.

The following situations could form the basis for discussion between you and your colleagues.

Situation 1 — Learning to be helpless

A newly admitted elderly woman is taken to the ward bathroom by a nurse. The woman tells the nurse: "Please don't worry. I can manage to get myself bathed on my own." "That's all right," says the nurse. "Here, let's run the water and get you undressed."

The elderly woman can interpret what has happened in a number of different ways. Look at the following possible interpretations and discuss the psychological effects of each one on future behaviour.

a) "I should have spoken up louder and really insisted on bathing myself."

b) "The nurses here just see the patients as pets to be looked after."

c) "Look at the state of me. I can't even get myself undressed and into the bath any more."

d) "I disliked that nurse the moment I saw her. She thinks she's the matron telling everyone what to do."

a) The woman is interpreting what happened to her on this occasion as resulting from a lack of effort on her part. It will probably lead her to take a more assertive stance on the next similar occasion. She has limited the damage to the specific event, but blames herself for lack of effort.

b) This interpretation is damaging in the sense that the woman has generalised from the behaviour of one nurse to that of all the nurses in the ward. However she is also attributing the fact that she did not get what she wanted to a source outside herself. It may lead to passive behaviour while on the ward, but she may continue to see herself as fully capable when discharged home.

c) This is the most damaging interpretation, and most likely to lead to helplessness and dependence. The woman internalises the fact that she has not got what she wanted, she interprets it as evidence of a permanent state of helplessness. It will usually take a whole series of adverse events to cause such a pessimistic interpretation, but nurses may have no idea of what has happened to new patients prior to admission.

d) This interpretation strongly reinforces the woman's view of herself as capable of influencing events. She attributes what happened to the nurse's bossy nature, and limits the problem to interactions with this particular nurse.

Situation 2 — Controlling language

The way a nurse talks to an elderly person may suggest that the nurse is in complete control and is offering the patient no choice in the matter. Frequently the words and the non-verbal communication are those of a parent to a child, rather than one adult to another.

Analyse the following sentences to find out which phrases emphasise the control exercised by the nurses. How could they be rephrased to achieve an adult-to-adult interchange?

a) "Now then Martin, lie on your side so that I can wash your bottom, there's a good chap."

b) "We'll just sit you down here in the day room."

c) "You will eat up all your dinner for me now, won't you?"

d) "Now don't you worry about what's going on at home. You just concentrate on getting better."

a) Try saying this aloud to hear the tone of voice that naturally accompanies the words. It is fine if Martin is six years old, but what if he's sixty-six? The use of the first name may not be appropriate, it depends on the relationship between the nurse and the patient. It could be rephrased as, "Please can you lie on your side so that I can wash your bottom."

b) The implication is that the patient's body is an object which the nurses move around at will. The word "just" is often used as a softener, when a nurse wants to do something to a patient without fully explaining it, or without giving any choice in the matter. An improved version might be, "We'll help you to sit down in the day room. Would you like to sit on this side of the room, or on the other side?" The phrasing shifts the nurses back into a helping role. Even if there is no choice about sitting in the day room, it is worth giving a limited choice on where to sit.

The other two examples can be analysed in the same way. It would help even the most experienced nurse to get an elderly patient's permission to tape record a conversation, and then listen to it for examples of the nurse using a patronising, "parent" tone of voice. It can be an enlightening experience!

Situation 3 — Regaining control

A communicating/counselling process can systematically help an elderly person to move towards a realistic view of themselves, through realising that there are still major areas over which the person can reasonably expect to exercise control.

A 70 year old woman whose husband died last year after a long illness complains to her health visitor that she cannot seem to talk to anyone in the village any more, which is why she now stays in the house as much as possible. Consider the following alternatives to the "Pull-yourself-together" approach to problem solving. Discuss the good points of each approach.

a) "You seemed to have a large circle of friends before your husband became ill. Would you say that people enjoyed your company then?"
b) "Next week when you go to the post office for your pension, give a smile and comment on the weather. Then we'll talk about what sort of response you got."
c) "You and I have talked a lot about what your husband meant to you, but other people could be afraid of upsetting you by mentioning him."
d) "You told me that your neighbours on the right always kept themselves to themselves, even while your husband was alive, but the woman across the road was very supportive when he was ill. How could you make contact with her again?"

a) Trying to help her to recognise that if she once had the capacity to maintain successful social relationships, she can probably do so again. She is encouraged to see her loneliness as being temporary.
b) Giving her graded tasks in which she is likely to be successful. Then encourage her to generalise from one success to the possibility of others, thus reversing the learning process.
c) Instead of attributing her loneliness to something in herself, she is encouraged to consider the possibility that part of the problem is external, due to the lack of understanding on the part of other people. Generally speaking an external attribution of failure is less damaging than an internal attribution.
d) Trying to help her to establish limited, realistic expectations of success and failure. Certainly, some people will not want to make contact, but others will be only too pleased to do so. The principle is one of changing an unrealistic global attribution of failure to a limited and specific one.

Situation 4 — When the person is disorientated

You are working in an assessment ward for the elderly mentally ill. As you wake up one patient and prepare to help him get dressed he reaches across the bed and says, "Where's my Elsie? Why isn't she in bed with me?" You know that Elsie, his wife, died last year before he was admitted to hospital.

Consider the following ways of handling the situation. What principles are illustrated in each, and on what basis could you decide which is the more suitable course of action?

a) "I think Elsie's already got up before you. Come on Mr Jones, why don't you get up too?"
b) "Now then Mr Jones, it's time to get up and come down to the ward dining room. Which shirt would you like to wear today?"
c) "You're in a hospital ward at the moment, Mr Jones. I remember that yesterday you were telling me about Elsie. Where did you say the two of you used to live?"
d) "I'm very sorry Mr Jones, but your wife died last year. This is a hospital you're in at the moment, not your own home."

a) Reinforcing the false belief, then using distraction. As a general rule (to which there are always exceptions) avoid this approach. It is important that if an elderly person is disorientated, the whole environment should be supportive, and all contacts should reinforce reality.
b) Distraction. If a person raises a subject which is likely to evoke a strong emotional reaction, the nurse needs to consider whether she can give enough time to this individual to help and support him through that reaction. It may be much the best course to distract the patient now, but give him another opportunity to talk about his wife later.
c) Emphasising reality in time and place, and encouraging the patient to go back to his intact long term memories and then gently work forward to the time of his wife's death. An adult approach, encouraging the patient to keep in touch with reality. Needs the right time and place. The nurse must understand the grieving process, and the likelihood of renewed trauma at rediscovering the death.
d) Reinforcing reality. It may be effective, it may also be cruel. The situation reveals the importance of assessing each patient individually. One suggestion is to try confronting the patient with reality when he is confused about something which is NOT emotionally charged — what was on the lunchtime menu for example. How does the patient react when he realises he has made a mistake? Even patients in the later stages of senile dementia may become frighteningly aware of the tragedy which has happened to them, and become severely depressed as well as demented.

Conclusion

All aspects of working with the elderly, particularly communication, demand great skill. Nurses can draw on research to guide them, and they themselves have a duty to develop their own body of applied research through evaluating the effects of their interventions.

Bibliography

Holden, U.P. and Woods, R. (1982) Reality Orientation. Churchill Livingstone, London.
Sound sense from authors who understand how to apply research to practice.
Hanley, I. and Hodge, J. (1984) Psychological Approaches to the Care of the Elderly. Croom Helm, London.
Includes detailed explanation of learned helplessness and how it may be overcome.
Lanceley, A. (1985) Use of controlling language in the rehabilitation of the elderly. Journal of Advanced Nursing, 10, 125-135.
A nurse opening up this area for future research.

Children's knowledge and understanding is based on their life experience, which is obviously very limited. This often makes them misconstrue things that seem patently obvious to adults. In the strange environment of the hospital, nurses must take great care to communicate clearly with children.

Communicating with children

June Jolly, SRN, RSCN

Until recently Co-ordinator, Child Health Services, Greenwich Health Authority

'Well, what's so different about that?'; 'I find them rather intimidating, don't you?'; 'They either ask impossible questions or start howling when you've only tried to explain what you are going to do.'; 'I don't know either, I can never get a sensible answer to the most elementary of questions.'

Such comments show why communicating with children must be taken seriously. Children's reasoning powers are commensurate with their mental and, frequently, physical age. Their understanding is limited not only by their vocabulary but also their life experience. The child who has grown up in the inner city will be more likely to be familiar with tubes and escalators — but try explaining what they are to an immigrant child, or one from the provinces or a very sheltered or deprived environment. When it comes to the child who needs hospital care, as a casualty, an out or in-patient, the task becomes more formidable. It is unlikely that anything will be familiar and the very strangeness of the environment added to pain or bewilderment will make it even more difficult to understand. The best way is to explain to the parent who can then interpret to the child. This, of course, is not always possible. Then a knowledge of the developmental processes which govern the child's increasing understanding and logical reasoning power will help.

For example — at six to seven months the baby recognises and shows fear of strangers. Aged one to three the toddler learns the meaning of 'No' and the power of using it and also becomes adventurous but has no sense of danger. Children under four rarely understand the concept of 'tomorrow' and, emotionally, relationships will be as they are to a mother. To 'go away' may imply 'never to come back'. Most children suffer from separation anxiety throughout the pre-school years, if parted from their parents.

Children under six are not always aware of their bodies as an integral part of themselves. But it is then they start to view an assault of one part as a threat to their whole being. Development of moral judgment and adult logical reasoning will not be complete until 10 to 12 years. It may still be confusing because the child has his own way of reasoning, and to slot into this may be the most helpful.

The following are real-life situations which could form the basis of discussion between yourself and colleagues.

Situation 1

Tim and Jenny had been admitted to their local hospital for tonsillectomy and were taken to the children's ward. The nurse told them about what would happen. She asked whether they knew where their tonsils were? Both pointed to their throats. She got them both to peer into each other's throats to see where they were. By putting out their tongues and panting like puppies they had a good view, and it was fun, too. She then explained about the magic sleep the doctor would give them — all very good. Asked how the doctor would get the tonsils out, Tim became very dubious. Using his index finger he took a quick slice across his throat from ear to ear and at the same time made a grimace. Jenny was horrified. Both children were between four and five.

How could the nurse reassure them that this barbaric procedure was not what would happen?

a) Give a simple straightforward explanation of the way the surgeon operated.

b) Use language and vocabulary with which the children were familiar to explain how their mouths could be opened whilst they were asleep.

c) Merely promise them they would be asleep and wouldn't feel anything.

Obviously the children would need explanation in terms they would understand. They also needed reassurance that they wouldn't be awake or feel anything. Sometimes in trying to be truthful we go into too much detail. Look at children's stories. They go into detail about very little, and then it is usually over the trivial or smaller issues. There is no need to give explanation about a procedure, but it is important to explain the things that worry the child.

Will they be sure to be asleep? How could they open their mouths — and would they stay open? How does the doctor get at the tonsils?

It is better to avoid using terms like scalpels, forceps, which they don't understand, or even knives or razors with which they might start experimenting later on their friends. A good plan is to describe events that the child will consciously remember. What he does not know will not normally matter to him. He will ask for information he wants. You do not need to do more than answer what he asks.

Situation 2

Philip aged six had orthopaedic surgery for correction of a congenital malformation of his leg, requiring a plaster cast. He was an only child of articulate parents who explained that the doctor would mend his leg so that he could play football like Daddy. He helped pack his nightclothes and chose some toys and games to take with him. His mother promised she would sleep there too and he was quite excited. In the ward the nurse showed him his bed and locker and introduced him to other children. He was told about the operation but it was not the custom to go into details of the surgery or to 'practise' wearing operation gowns etc. After surgery he appeared to make a good recovery. Next day however this usually chatty West Indian boy was silent. Even his parents could not get him to speak and he remained withdrawn for several weeks, making them feel he was blaming them and couldn't trust them anymore.

What clues are there to help 'get inside his mind' to see what the trouble was?

a) Why might Philip have felt he was being punished? What sort of things do parents say inadvertently?

b) Had he been let down by this hospitalisation? What might his family have neglected to tell him?

c) Had the plaster of paris on his leg been what he had expected and what did it mean?

a) and b) It is unlikely that having been prepared by his mother and the hospital staff that he really felt he was being 'punished'. The fact that his mother stayed with him should have alleviated any anxiety that this had happened because he wasn't loved.

c) Children of this age do not always understand things in an adult fashion. Whereas an adult may wonder how a hard plaster of paris could be removed, children may assume it is a permanent alternative limb. If this was compounded by the shock of finding it white, he could well have been shocked. A good way of teaching children about plaster of paris casts is to let them help put a small one on a favourite doll or model. By cutting it off with scissors after it had hardened, gives a child much more confidence that this could and will happen, than any amount of explaining.

Situation 3

Julie aged seven had been in hospital for a few days with a severe infection for which she needed antibiotics. On the third day she objected strongly to the injection so the nurse said 'don't worry, I'll give it by mouth instead'. The child became hysterical. Why? She misinterpreted the nurse and thought she would be given the injection into her mouth. How could the nurse have made sure she understood and was reassured?

a) Explained that the alternative way of giving the medicine was in a syrup which she could swallow.

b) Shown her the medicine and the measure or spoon. Discuss other ways in which the child might have been reassured and not terrified.

This is a good example of a child's 'defective' understanding. No adult would have imagined that an injection would be given into the mouth. By mouth is well understood by adults. But why should children have this knowledge? There are many illustrations that could be given for this sort of misunderstanding. Any explanation needs to be carefully worded and preferably accompanied by a visual aid, either on yourself, another adult (Mummy for preference) or a doll.

Situation 4

Barry, aged five, had been diagnosed as having a defect in his heart. His family had an open and positive attitude towards Barry's difficulty. One day he asked his mother — 'Will I be able to love when I grow up?'.

His mother asked him, 'Why do you think you won't be able to love?' to which he replied, 'Well I've got something wrong with my heart so I thought I couldn't.'

How would you have answered his question? Do you think that would have elicited the reply the mother got?

The principle of reflecting a question is even more valid with children than with adults. When a child asks what appears to be a 'stupid' or obtuse question it is worth finding out what he really means before coming in with a trite answer.

The words in the box are taken at random from the ward furniture. Among yourselves try to explain what each item is so that a child would understand its use.

Bed table	Suction machine	Monkey pole
Traction	Suction catheter	Patella hammer
Oxygen tent	Incubator	Bedpan/bottle
Bed cradle	Syringe driver	Operation gown

Now look at the words again and try to imagine what a child might think you meant when hearing you use it initially. This will give you a good insight into how children can so easily get the 'wrong end of the stick.'

Bibliography

Donaldson, M. (1978) Children's Minds. Fontana/Collins, London. A new approach to Piaget's theory of development.

McLeod Clark, J. and Bridge, W. (1981) Communication in Nursing Care. HM&M, Aylesbury. Includes a chapter on communication.

Petrillo M. and Sangers, S. (1980) Emotional Care of Hospitalised Children. Lippincott, Philadelphia. Definitive work on communicating with children and meeting their emotional needs.

Rodin, J. (1983) Does it hurt? RCN Monograph. Research on children's concepts of hospital and medical tests and their need to be prepared.

Jolly, J. (1981) The Other Side of Paediatrics. Macmillan Education, Basingstoke. Meeting the every day needs of children who have to be in hospital.

People requiring hospital care are often extremely anxious, whether their illness is serious or not. How can nurses learn to recognise and deal with anxious patients individually?

Giving reassurance to anxious patients

Kevin Teasdale, MA, Cert Ed, RMN
Director of In-Service Training and Post Basic Nurse Education, Pilgrim Hospital, Boston, Lincs.

How often in your nurse training were you told to "reassure the patient"? How many times did you write "give reassurance" in an examination answer in order to prove that you had considered the patient's psychological needs? To really help a person feel more calm and in control depends on far more complex knowledge and skills than bland statements about reassurance suggest.

It is important in considering reassurance to concentrate on the effect the nurse's actions have on the patient, rather than to think of the actions in isolation. Ask the question — is the patient now more calm, balanced and relaxed than before? If so, reassurance has been given. There is no such thing as a single skill, "giving reassurance", which can be learned and will be effective in all situations.

The following situations use the framework of the nursing process as a stimulus for discussion.

1. Assessing coping styles
Individuals cope with stress and anxiety in various ways, even when the precipitating threat is the same for each. Imagine four people just admitted to hospital for a major operation. Consider the following ways in which each person might try to cope with the anxiety. How would you describe each coping style, and what are the consequences of each for the person's preoperative preparation and postoperative recovery?
a. "No, I'm not worried about a thing. It's only a minor operation."
b. "Can you tell me what a 'pre-med' is, and what it's for?"
c. "I'm feeling a little sick at the moment. Please will you stay with me?"
d. "It's all right for you nurses sitting there writing up care plans. You ought to spend less time talking about care and more time doing it."

a. Denial. The person is making light of the operation and wants others to adopt the same attitude. A person using this coping style will actively discourage others from giving information about the operation, or how he might feel afterwards. People who do not have a realistic understanding of postoperative pain may find this especially frightening.
b. Seeking information. The person is trying to prepare psychologically by finding out exactly what will happen. When the events occur, they may be less anxiety-provoking because they have already been mentally rehearsed.
c. Dependence. The person is trying to draw strength and comfort from the nurse as a young child will seek protection and safety from parents. Nurses and doctors can use this to calm and comfort people. However the comforting needs to be tempered with realism. If the patient suffers more pain or discomfort than expected, they may come to be seen as punishing "parents" instead.
d. Aggression. Attack is said to be the best form of defence. This patient tries to mask gnawing fear by using anger, which is easily misunderstood, leading to his being left isolated and unprepared.

2. Planning how to act
It is important for nurses to become skilled in identifying a whole range of coping styles, and adapting their plans to the patient's chosen style and their analysis of its possible consequences, given the situation in which the patient finds himself.

Consider this nursing care plan. Discuss how each section is in its own way inadequate, and how each might be improved.

a. Problem — the patient is anxious about having a barium enema.
b. Goal — for the patient to feel calm and prepared for the barium enema.
c. Action — reassure the patient.
d. Evaluation record — procedure explained. Patient taken to X-ray and barium enema given.

a. The problem is not described in enough detail. Is it the procedure about which the patient is anxious, or fear of the results? Improvement involves an accurate description of the source of anxiety, and how the patient is trying to cope.
b. How will the nurse know if the patient is feeling calm and prepared? Goals are easier to evaluate if they describe what the patient will say or do.
c. "Reassure" is not sufficiently specific. Does it mean telling the patient not to worry? Will the person be reassured by full explanation of the procedure, or will it make him more anxious? Research suggests the former, but if his main coping style is denial then explanation may be rejected. Will it help simply to listen and allow the patient to express his fears? The intervention selected will depend on the initial assessment.
d. Evaluation is more than a commentary on what a nurse has done. It means looking first at the patient's goal and considering whether it has been achieved. If not, it means making changes to the plan of care. Often the problem of anxiety is crossed out as soon as the feared procedure has taken place. But in many cases the coping style used by the patient will affect recovery physically and psychologically. The plan must be developed to take this into account.

3. Implementing the plan

A patient suffering from lung cancer is being treated with radiotherapy. She has been told her diagnosis but has not referred to it since, or seemed interested in the details of her treatment. However she has talked to nurses about what she will do once she is "back to normal", and has cooperated fully in her treatment. Recently she appears very tired and withdrawn. The care plan, which is kept at the bedside, refers to the potential problem of her treatment making her feel tired and discouraged. The goal is for her to talk about how she feels, and to ask questions about anything she is unsure of. The prescribed nursing action is to support her chosen coping style, allow opportunities to talk, and give any information she wants.

Her primary nurse is off duty and you are acting as associate nurse. The patient looks at herself in the mirror and says to you: "I'm scared. Why am I so much thinner and paler than last week? What's happening to me? Am I going to die?" Which of the following actions are in keeping with the prescribed plan of care? What factors would make you select one in preference to another?

a. "Don't be so silly. What you need is a new mirror. Now, let's get your make-up on, you'll soon feel brighter."
b. "I can see you're frightened and you feel you're not as well as you were before. Is it something you've been thinking for some time?"
c. "The radiotherapy will make you tired and your appetite will suffer. Am I right in thinking that sometimes you wonder whether it's making you better or worse?"
d. Holding her hand — "You know we all die sometime. The important thing is to live every day to the full."

a. This statement supports someone who is using denial as a coping style. The problem with denial comes when a person's condition changes for the worse, so that it becomes harder to deny the reality of the change. By talking about her fear, the woman is signalling that she needs to find a new coping style. The nurse's reply tries to force her back into denial, and cuts off further discussion. It may be that denial is the way the nurse herself copes with the stress of nursing someone suffering from cancer.

b. Acknowledging the patient's feelings, and encouraging her to talk. Some would criticise an open approach like this. The patient may decide to give up fighting and instead try to cope with what she sees as the certain prospect of death. Her clinical condition may or may not justify this decision. The acceptability of the nurse's response will depend on the model of nursing used by the team, particularly as regards the rights of patients to information and autonomy.

c. Similar to b. in encouraging the patient to talk. It gives the patient information about radiotherapy, and implies that the patient's fears about death are misplaced. If the information is accurate and the nurse is not too directive, then the approach is sound. Very often, however, the clinical condition of the patient is unclear. In such circumstances should one always encourage hope, even at the risk of one's predictions being found to be inaccurate? The present state of nursing research offers no definite answer. But at least as a nurse one can consider the problem consciously and make explicit one's own philosophy of care under these circumstances.

d. Uses sympathy and touch to try to guide the patient away from open consideration of her possible death. The reply is conventionally "reassuring" but may not encourage the patient to talk about her feelings as the care plan prescribes.

4. Evaluating the results

Assume that the nurse in the previous example selected option c. — explaining the effects of radiotherapy, but allowing the woman to talk further about how she feels. Consider which of these four possible reactions suggest that the nurse's intervention was found "reassuring" and which suggest that it was not.

a. The patient replies that she has been feeling this way for several weeks now but somehow couldn't admit it to herself or to anyone else.
b. The patient dissolves in tears, but does not answer the nurse's question.
c. She replies as in the first answer, and appears calmer after talking for a while with the nurse. At visiting time her relatives report that she seems quiet and remote.
d. She reacts as in a., and at the next ward round asks the consultant to give her a full explanation of radiotherapy and her chances of benefiting from it.

a. The reply suggests that the woman has accepted the opportunity given by the nurse to explore her worries and fears more openly. She may be reassured by being able to talk with and seek support from someone else.

b. Tears are often misinterpreted as necessarily being the unsatisfactory result of inept handling of a situation by a nurse. Frequently they indicate a release of tension. It may be possible to help this patient to learn from her pain, and develop more effective ways of coping. This will depend on the nurse's full assessment of the situation. Too often automatic "reassurance" is given, perhaps to save nurses from their own distress rather than to help the patient.

c. It is unrealistic to expect a patient who is trying to come to terms with her fears of pain, discomfort and possible death to do so on the basis of one short talk with a nurse. In formal counselling much of the "work" is done by the client in between the sessions with the counsellor. The same will be true in the less structured, but no less valid interactions between nurse and patient. The relatives' observation means the nurses must continue to give the patient opportunities to talk, and support her without forcing themselves on her.

d. This suggests that the woman may have decided that denial as a coping strategy is no longer effective in warding off her anxiety. She is trying to move to a more open understanding and awareness of her condition. All members of the team need to understand this in order to support her effectively.

Conclusion

Reassurance is a state of restored calmness or equilibrium in the patient, which MAY or MAY NOT result from nursing actions. It is vital to focus on the effects of one's actions, rather than on the caring intention alone. Viewed in this way, an action such as giving information is not "reassuring" in itself. It depends on the accuracy of one's assessment, the logic and flexibility of one's plan of action, and the skills used in implementing it. Even then, only accurate and continuing evaluation will allow the nurse to state — "I reassured the patient."

Bibliography

Bridge, W. and Macleod Clark, J. (Eds) (1981) Communication in Nursing Care. John Wiley & Sons, Chichester.
A good overview of nursing research. The chapter by Maggie Hacking on dying patients is outstanding.
French, H.P. (1979) Reassurance: a nursing skill? Journal of Advanced Nursing, 4, 627-34.
Weinman, J. (1981) An Outline of Psychology as applied to Medicine. John Wiley & Sons, Bristol.
Chapter five is a general introduction to theories of stress and coping styles.

If patients comply with medical advice, intervention will be more effective. However, they must be given enough information to enable them to understand their instructions, which is the responsibility of health care staff.

Compliance: a shared responsibility

Ruth E. Smith, BSc, RGN, DNCert.
Support Worker in Rehabilitation, Lothian Regional Council, Department of Social Work

Jill Birrell, MA(Hons), MSc, AFBPs, CPsychol
Principal Clinical Psychologist, Royal Edinburgh Hospital

When we use the term 'compliance' we usually refer to adherence or co-operation on the part of the patient in following a health care professional's advice with regard to health related behaviours.

It is interesting to note however that we all comply in various ways in everyday life. Most people comply with the law, health professionals comply with hospital policy and usually with instructions and directions from their immediate managers. We all generally comply with unwritten social rules.

Ley (1981) reported that health care professionals do not always follow the best available recommendations when treating patients (an 80 per cent non-compliance rate) and that on 65 per cent of occasions the medication and advice they give is not appropriate.

If we combine this information with the reasons patients give regarding dissatisfaction with the health care they receive then the rates of non-compliance recorded in research studies are hardly surprising.

Despite this information, non-compliance seems to be blamed on the patient's 'unco-operative personality' although there is no research evidence to support this.

Below are several situations in which the nurse involved may influence the likelihood of compliance. Situations 1, 2 and 3 deal with the issue of patient compliance, as this is the area which nurses deal with most frequently. Situation 4, which focuses on staff compliance, is included to emphasise the fact that certain principles apply regardless of the groups of people involved, and also that compliance is not only restricted to patients.

Situation 1
You are visiting Mrs. Smith, a 45 year old lady with insulin dependent diabetes, at home. Mrs. Smith has had three admissions to hospital in the past year due to instability of her condition. Her general practitioner has asked you to become involved and the evidence seems to suggest she is not following medical advice at home.

How would you approach Mrs. Smith?
a) Confront her with the evidence that she is not complying with advice.
b) Go in routinely to supervise urine testing, her insulin injections and diet.
c) Ignore the evidence surrounding Mrs. Smith's non-compliance and try to build up a relationship of trust with her.
d) Visit Mrs. Smith regularly but with the focus being on how she is managing generally.

The overall aim of your involvement is to discover how Mrs. Smith is coping with her illness at home. Confronting Mrs. Smith may give you that information. On the other hand Mrs. Smith may simply refuse to see you again. Supervising urine testing, insulin injections and diet only allows you to make 'spot checks' and may not give you a picture of what is happening at other times. It is important however, early on in your involvement, to supervise these tasks as Mrs. Smith may not be carrying them out correctly, either because she has not been taught correctly or she has forgotten. A relationship of trust is important and this may allow Mrs. Smith to discuss any difficulties with you — visits may however develop into 'social chat' which does not give you the information you require and may allow another episode of instability to occur.

Allowing Mrs. Smith time to talk about how she is managing at home may hopefully elicit information that lets you understand the problem she is facing in following medical advice — it does however involve a frequent commitment of time. Within this framework, there may be times when social chat or even confrontation seems appropriate. If it is not possible to allocate the time you feel is required, report this back to the general practitioner and your nurse manager.

Situation 2

You are working in a rehabilitation ward for psychiatric patients. It is well documented that psychiatric patients, particularly those on long term medication, risk a recurrence of their illness by not complying with medication. You decide to try and improve compliance. What do you do?

a) Make available written information regarding non-compliance and the risk of recurrence of illness.

b) Introduce a trial period of self medication prior to discharge.

c) Spend time individually with each patient trying to discover what questions they have regarding this.

d) Start a ward programme giving talks on why medication is important.

e) Arrange for each patient to be visited at home after discharge.

It is important to spend time with each patient discussing with them what problems they envisage. Patients may not understand the importance of medication, particularly if they feel 'well'. Written information is only useful if it can be understood and if it answers the questions an individual has. Handouts, if they are used, should have the information well laid out and categorised. Instructions should be given in specific terms, eg 'take medication once a day' rather than 'regularly'. 'Set talks' can only cover general principles — time must be taken to ensure they are understood and that they are covering the information required. A home visit after discharge may be helpful but if the patient has left the ward with questions unanswered or with mistaken beliefs intact then this might not be recognised on one visit. This is particularly true if the visit is not carried out by ward staff. A trial period of self medication is valuable if this can be arranged. It is easy to remember to take medication if a nurse calls you at the correct time and hands you the correct tablets.

Situation 3

Miss Jones, age 56, is undergoing radiotherapy for metastasis following a mastectomy two years previously. Miss Jones had also been prescribed chemotherapy which she had been taking regularly prior to her admission to the oncology ward. One evening Miss Jones asks to see you in your position as staff nurse. She informs you of her decision not to accept any further radiotherapy or chemotherapy. How do you respond?

a) Agree promptly and avoid any discussion.

b) Tell her to discuss her decision with medical staff.

c) Agree to discuss the matter later but don't.

d) Try to persuade Miss Jones to change her mind.

e) Listen to her reasons and agree to discuss it with the ward team.

f) Ask another member of staff to speak to her.

Unless you genuinely feel you have neither the time required or the necessary skill it is important to discuss Miss Jones' decision with her. If you do have to involve another member of staff then this member of staff must feel competent to deal with the situation. The reasons for involving someone else must be explained to Miss Jones. It is important to listen to the reasons/beliefs behind her decision as it may be lack of knowledge or incorrect assumptions that have led to the decision. If, after discussion, Miss Jones appears to have reached her decision based on correct information available then it is important to respect it as her decision — this is not the same as agreeing with it. To deny Miss Jones the opportunity for discussion or to deny her right to make that decision is to deny her importance as an individual. Keep channels of communication open with Miss Jones and discuss her decision with other members of the ward team including medical staff.

Situation 4

You have moved to your first sister's post. You believe that certain of the practices carried out are not those most beneficial to the patient. You start to initiate changes but find yourself meeting opposition particularly from senior members of the ward team. To comply with what seems to be expected of you by both medical and nursing staff does not appear to you to be in the best interest of the patient. What do you do?

a) Speak to your nurse manager.

b) Continue making changes hoping they will become accepted.

c) Seek out other charge nurses/sisters for support.

d) Decide to leave the situation as it is.

e) Ask for a transfer to another ward.

There are certain steps you should have taken before initiating any changes — the most important being discussion with those who will be required to implement them. Changes which involve the overall running of the ward or hospital policy should also have been discussed with nurse management. If you insist on changes without discussion or explanation of the reasoning behind them then it is possible they may only be carried out when you are on duty and even then grudgingly. You need to sit down with other members of the ward team and discuss what you want to change and why — equally you need to listen to their reasons for resisting these changes. To insist on compliance without discussion leads to a stifling of initiative in others and may denote an individual who is insecure in their position and wishes to retain power. Leaving the situation as it is or asking for a transfer does not improve the care received by the patients. Getting support from other charge nurses/sisters may help by allowing you to discuss the problem and also benefit from their experience.

Summary

For a patient to comply with medical advice, he must have the knowledge to understand that advice, the capabilities to carry it out and accept that it is important for him to do so.

If we continue to view compliance as the sole responsibility of the patient, we deny ourselves the opportunity of changing the rates of non-compliance reported. It is only by seeing compliance in terms of a shared responsibility between health care professionals and clients that we may utilise our skills in this area.

References

Ley, P. (1981) 'Professional Non-Compliance: A Neglected Problem'. *British Journal of Clinical Psychology*, **20**, 151-154.

Terminally ill patients who are also mentally confused pose special problems for those caring for them. How can nurses assess and deal with each individual patient?

Mental confusion in the dying patient

Sue Hawkett, RGN, RSCN, SCM, DipN, Cert Ed, MSc
Senior Tutor, St Mary's School of Nursing, London

In caring for the terminally ill it is distressing to see patients who are sometimes anxious, depressed or suffering from mental confusion. Much can be done to control painful symptoms, and psychological pain is often relieved, but mental confusion in the dying patient is recognised by many authorities in continuing or terminal care as being to some extent an unresolved and difficult problem.

Confusion is frequently a vague and unhelpful term used to describe a variety of symptoms and situations meaning different things to different people. Walton (1985) describes confusion as "impairment of consciousness with lack of mental processes short of stupor or coma", when discussing diseases of the central nervous system. Twycross and Lack (1984), considering confusion in patients with advanced cancer, describe it as a mental state marked by the mingling of ideas, which results in them experiencing bewilderment and disturbance of comprehension.

Patients who are near to death often suffer from a variety of disturbing experiences commonly referred to as confusion. However, within the so-called confusion there often lurks a rational and lucid explanation which should be sought and listened for.

It is important to try to make some sense out of what might appear to be the disorientated ramblings of a very sick person, and to seek the causative agent. The effects of drugs, biochemical and metabolic disturbances, brain tumour or brain secondaries and the psychological stress related to dying should all be carefully considered (Stedeford, 1984).

The nurse's response is so often coloured by the pressure to control the situation because of the disruptive influence of the confused patient. However, at the heart of good nursing practice lies the willingness to understand the patient, to listen for the feeling behind the words and to combine knowledge of the disease process and of the person with sensitivity and insight. It can be frightening for a patient to be partly aware of what is happening and to think he is losing his mind.

It is important that the nurse should always assume a patient understands, and recognise that confusion is frightening for the patient, and that it is usually treatable and manageable (Regnard, 1983).

The following situations could form the basis for discussion between you and your colleagues.

---

1. The rights of the patient

Mrs James is 76 years old, uraemic and described as confused. She is rambling, disorientated and behaving inappropriately. The nurse manages to carry out a rectal examination and assesses that she needs glycerine suppositories. As the nurse prepares to insert them Mrs James clearly announces "Don't do that, don't do that, go away!" What action should the nurse take?
a. Insist that she does need them.
b. Consider an oral aperient.
c. Ensure Mrs James drinks more fluids.
d. Leave her and offer a commode later.

a. Here is a dilemma of a patient's right to be treated as an adult and to be in control, versus professional judgement regarding treatment. However, Mrs James's agitation may be exacerbated if it becomes an issue which requires professional force.
b. Choosing an aperient that both softens faeces and stimulates peristalic action may overcome the problem.
c. This will mean the nurse spending longer with Mrs James and may give helpful insight into her behaviour. Mrs James may refuse to drink.
d. If she was being rational, this would test it out.

---

2. Sudden distress

Miss Samuel is in a room opposite the ward kitchen. Suddenly she becomes very agitated and upset, crying out "Poor Kath, they are killing her!" It is noticed that her distress coincides with the liquidiser being used. How can Miss Samuel be helped?
a. (i) Use the liquidiser out of earshot, or (ii) move her bed to a quieter area.
b. Ask about Kath and talk to the family.
c. Consider sedation.

a. An immediate and practical solution: (i) would remove the trigger for her confused response but not the underlying reason; (ii) moving her bed may disorientate her, or make her feel she had been punished for bad behaviour.
b. Understanding more about her background and family may uncover an unresolved grief or guilt not previously expressed.
c. Careful sedation would relax her and relieve anxiety.

3. The dominant coper

Mrs Brown is middle-aged and has advanced cancer of the ovary, with pelvic involvement and liver metastasis. She has been admitted for control of her painful symptoms. She is described as a dominant coper, someone who had always been in control. Now she is anxious, suspicious and frightened. She constantly paces around the ward in obvious pain and distress, telling each nurse that she has had a drink of water and that she has taken her tablets. Her anxiety and distress increase and she begins to resist all physical care. She cries during the night but will not talk about her fears.

Consider the following questions:
a. What drugs are being given? Are they appropriate?
b. Should an opportunity for a conversation be initiated?
c. Should a family meeting with the patient take place?

a. Mrs Brown's drug regime needs to be scrutinised by the nursing and medical staff and the following considered carefully:
  i. Is she receiving the appropriate drugs for her agitation and anxiety? As she does not appear to be hallucinating or suffering from a psychosis, an anxiolytic which would also sedate might be considered.
  ii. Are any antagonists inadvertently being used, or is Mrs Brown having an idiosyncratic response to one of the drugs?
  iii. Is she receiving inadequate analgesia, so that pain is exacerbating her agitation?
  iv. Is she receiving the right combination and dose of phenothiazine and analgesic?

b. Mrs Brown needs her distressing physical symptoms to be controlled before she will be able to respond to counselling. The nurse will then be able to engage in non-directive counselling in an attempt to discover what Mrs Brown is frightened of. Opening statements such as "You appear to be very worried and unhappy, Mrs Brown" may facilitate a conversation. A combination of being both pain-free and relaxed is necessary to encourage her to talk. It is important to listen carefully, without feeling pressure to say or do anything.

c. A family meeting may be the most productive action in understanding the confusion and fear of a patient. Often it is the key to treatment and management. Through such meetings, ideally with other members of the caring team and the patient, the family is helped to understand the disease process, and the family helps the carers to understand the patient. It also provides an opportunity for the family to express its affection and sorrow to the patient.

4. Resisting help

Mr Roberts is 80 years old and has cancer of the bronchus. He has a chest infection and is anoxic, muddled and agitated. As the nurse washes him he thrashes about in his bed and resists all attempts to make him comfortable. The nurse eventually gives up and sits quietly beside him and Mr Roberts slowly becomes calm. What should she do next?
a. Attempt to wash him again.
b. Assess ways of relieving his distressing symptoms.
c. Explore quietly with him how he is feeling and what anxieties he has.

a. After a rest he may be ready to be washed and if the nurse has spent some time sitting with him he may not see it as an 'attack'.
b. This is probably the key. The chest infection and anoxia may be compounding his confusion.
c. Anxiety and fear are very real and exacerbate confusion. Acknowledging and allowing expression of these feelings in combination with (b) may help the confusion to subside.

Conclusion

Confusion is frightening and most of us dread 'losing our minds'. In the examples given there was always a lucid or rational part to the situation. Identifying this and acknowledging it can bring a degree of calm to patient, family and staff.

References

Walton, J. (Ed) (1985) Brain's diseases of the nervous system. Ninth edition. Oxford Medical Publications, Oxford.
Regnard, C. (1983) Confusional states. Paper presented at Cancer Relief Seminar, ''Maintaining Standards''. Abingdon.
Stedeford, A. (1984) Facing Death. Heinemann, London.
Twycross, R. and Lack, S. (1984) Therapeutics in Terminal Cancer. Pitman, Bath.

To enable accurate assessment and treatment of the patient in pain, effective communication between the caring team, the patient and the family is essential. But do we as nurses, in the highly pressurised environment in which we work, practise effective communication when caring for patients in chronic pain?

Management of pain: good communication

Jane Latham, SRN, DN

Senior Nurse, Pain Relief Unit, King's College Hospital, London

Each person's perception of pain is influenced by many different physical, psychological, social and environmental factors. Assessment and management of the patient's pain is facilitated by good communication. This Practice Check gives you an opportunity to explore this and to assess your own practice.

What can happen? Some ideas of what can happen between the patient, the patient's family and the therapeutic team when good and bad communication and practice take place are set out in Figures 1 and 2. These will be useful as "thought provokers" while considering and discussing the three hypothetical case histories. It may also be useful to carry out similar practice checks, on patients in pain within your clinical situation.

The following situations can form the basis for discussion between yourself and colleagues.

Situation 1

Mrs Andrews is 40 and is on an orthopaedic ward following an episode of acute chronic low back pain. No major cause has been found. She is extremely difficult to manage as she is reluctant to exercise and demands p.r.n. analgesia despite regular non-steroidal anti-inflammatory drugs and moderate analgesics. Transcutaneous nerve stimulation (TCNS) gives some relief. Mr Andrews visits daily with the two children, who want to know when their mother is coming home.

What should be done?

a) Discharge Mrs Andrews home on her present medication and follow up with appropriate out-patients clinics.

b) Discharge her on a different combination of drugs and follow up in appropriate out-patient clinics.

c) Discuss the patient and family with Mr Andrews without involving her.

d) While Mrs Andrews is having her TCNS treatment encourage her to talk about her pain, her family and any other anxieties she may have. Offer appropriate support and follow up as needed.

a) & b) are actions that occur frequently, but only offer an answer to the physical cause of the pain.

c) may cause a barrier between Mrs Andrews, her family and the therapeutic team, if she realises her treatment is being discussed without her involvement and agreement.

d) offers not only an answer to the physical pain, but also gives vital time to discuss and offer support to social/psychological pressures which can exacerbate such a chronic situation.

Situation 2

Mr Bates is 70 years old and has had a routine repair of an ingroinal hernia. When the nurses and physiotherapists tried to mobilise him on the third day after his operation he complained of acute pain. Analgesics were given. His recovery appears to have been uncomplicated. Mrs Bates visits regularly, and appears to be very concerned.

What should be done?

a) Stop the injections and insist that Mr Bates can manage on oral analgesic.

b) Carry on with the physiotherapy, mobilisation and home plans despite the protests from Mr Bates.

c) Discuss the situation with Mr and Mrs Bates together, arrange discharge with appropriate support.

d) Discuss the situation with Mr and Mrs Bates separately.

We need to establish the reasons for Mr Bates' continuing pain. **a) & b)** do not achieve this and the routine they represent simply reinforces the lack of effective communication between the nurses and their patient.

c) Seeing Mr and Mrs Bates together may not enable either of them to express their anxiety about the situation; it isn't always easy to talk about someone when they are there.

d) is more likely to identify all the problems which clearly underly this situation. This approach could be followed by joint discussion with Mr and Mrs Bates.

Situation 3

Mrs Curtis is an 80 year old widow who has been complaining of acute pain in addition to her extensive history of chronic non-specific aches and pains. Both kinds of pain vary in position and description from month to month. Routine investigations have shown no abnormalities to correlate with the presentations. Minor arthritic changes have been treated with non steroidal anti-inflammatory drugs.

The district nurse has been to call to assess if there is anything she can offer to assist Mrs Curtis, as she has been complaining of being unable to wash herself because of the pain, and had appeared quite unkempt.

What should be done?

a) Refer Mrs Curtis to social services assessment for day care and home help.

b) At a weekly staff meeting delegate the task of giving Mrs Curtis a weekly bath to one of the nursing auxilliaries.

c) Monitor Mrs Curtis's medications and persuade her to carry on on her own with only monthly support.

d) Continue to make visits form supervision of general care and refer, as appropriate, to other disciplines after further in-depth assessment.

a) & b) Immediately refer Mrs Curtis on to social workers or non-professional help which will not investigate or evaluate her clinical condition further.

c) will still involve the district nurse but time will not be available for her to talk about her problems on a monthly visit. She is therefore left to cope with her own condition.

d) will allow time for total nursing assessment of the patient during which time the problems underlying her condition should hopefully be identified. These could include bereavement. Once the nature of the problem is known an appropriate strategy for referral or intervention can be drawn up.

Figure 1. Problems that can result from bad communication and practice.

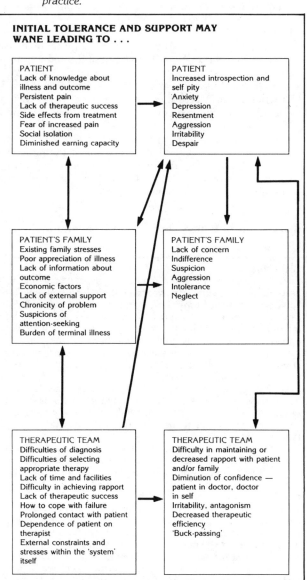

Figure 2. The benefits of good communication and practice.

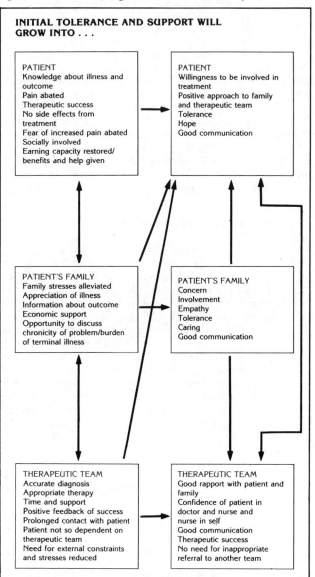

The grief of each individual takes a different form and proceeds at a different rate. Nurses will encounter grief in their patients, patients' relatives, colleagues, and in themselves, and with a knowledge and understanding of the process of grieving are better prepared to provide counselling and support.

Recognising grief

Julie Barnard, SEN, Diploma in Counselling
Enrolled Nurse, Brighton General Hospital

Grief is the normal process by which individuals adjust and adapt to accept a significant loss in their lives. The loss they experience may result from the death of, or separation from, a close friend or relative; from the loss of a valued object or possession; or from a change in their own pattern of life, for example as a result of losing a job, or a change in their own health, perhaps resulting in loss of mobility, sight, hearing, or of self-image, or even as a result of realising that they are dying and that the most significant change in life-style is about to take place.

Each individual's experience of grief is different, as is the time scale for the grieving process which cannot be hurried. However, various stages can be identified in grieving (Kubler-Rose, 1969) and we need to recognise these in order to provide understanding and support. An individual will not necessarily pass through these stages in sequence; he may return to earlier stages along the way.
Denial: This stage allows the person to mobilise his defences. He may avoid talking about the subject of death or loss, and particularly avoid discussing the truth about his own illness with his family by changing the subject or walking away, and often withdrawing into himself.
Anger: The individual often experiences anger that he should be the one chosen: "Why me?". The anger is often projected into the environment and towards immediate family or caring staff.
Bargaining: In this stage the individual tries to postpone death and extend his life with promises of good behaviour.
Depression: Gradually the person begins to withdraw and to prepare himself for the final separation. This is often the most traumatic stage for relatives, friends, and carers.
Acceptance: This is the final stage, in which the person is able to meet death peacefully. It can be almost euphoric, as the person becomes detached from interests and feelings.

These stages will also be experienced by members of the family and friends, although not at the same time as the dying person.

The most valuable response to a person in grief is that of listening and accepting without judgement, and of encouraging the person to express their feelings. Platitudes and attempts to provide everyday answers to the person's questions are of no value. To take on this listening role, the counsellor must be able to examine their own feelings, and will need the support of caring colleagues. No one should try to carry on alone and unsupported in this counselling role.

The following situations could form the basis for discussion between yourself and colleagues

1. Nurse Smith is newly qualified and has shown considerable ability in caring and communicating effectively with patients. Mr. Jones is admitted for major surgery while she is on duty. She shows considerable insight into his fears and anxieties. Immediately prior to surgery she has no problem helping him come to terms with his forthcoming operation. During operation it is discovered that Mr. Jones has a large inoperable tumour and palliative surgery is performed. Following the initial two days of post-operative recovery Nurse Smith, with the supervision of a staff nurse, is looking after Mr. Jones. It is then that the staff nurse notices that Nurse Smith's attitude to the patient has changed. She now fails to maintain eye contact, she seems withdrawn and irritable and becomes easily upset. Nurse Smith reveals to one of her colleagues that she finds the thought of death difficult to deal with. This information is relayed to the staff nurse concerned.

   How in a counselling situation can the staff nurse help Nurse Smith to discover what is happening to her? Should she:

   a) Tell Nurse Smith to "pull herself together" and say "If I were you I would . . ."?

Situation 1
   a) This sort of statement is of little value. It is wrong to assume that everyone can overcome their distress simply by "pulling themselves together". What is needed is for Nurse Smith to be allowed to express what she feels and not to be inhibited by the situation. It is not helpful for personal growth and development to rely on the suggestions of other people. To answer Nurse Smith in this way would merely make her suppress her emotions and feelings. The counsellor should remain non-judgemental and non-moralistic.
   b) Everything will not be alright. Reassurance has its place and it may help Nurse Smith to be told that her feelings are understandable and acceptable, but the situation is obviously a cause for concern, and the staff nurse needs to find out why Nurse Smith is acting in this way.
   c) If Nurse Smith is offered the time and concern of a caring colleague, and is encouraged to talk about her feelings, she will be able to understand and perhaps come to terms with her own experience of grief for the patient. Counselling can only be effective if the client wishes it to be and if the person taking on the task sees it as part of her role. It may take several sessions before Nurse Smith can come to terms with her problem. In doing so, deeply hidden feelings may be revealed which can cause the nurse a great deal of emotional distress. It may be that she has unresolved personal grief, anticipated loss of a parent or husband, or fear of her own death. The staff nurse needs to act in such a way that these fears may

b) Give reassurance, and tell Nurse Smith that everything will be alright?

c) Encourage Nurse Smith to talk about her feelings?

be expressed fully. Careful listening, showing empathy, and getting in touch with one's own feelings, play a large part in the art of counselling. Nurse Smith may also feel that confidentiality is of prime importance. The staff nurse cannot promise that absolutely: there may be circumstances in which she may need to discuss Nurse Smith's problems with another colleague, but she can reassure Nurse Smith of confidentiality within their immediate group, and that she would consult her before discussing her problems with anyone else.

---

2. Mr. Thomas is 60 years old and is dying from terminal cancer. When first told his diagnosis Mr. Thomas seemed distant and unable to talk about his illness. He withdrew into himself and refused to see his family. He was distrustful of staff and other patients alike but despite this would often be seen acknowledging their presence by waving to them, or explaining to nurses how good he was at eating his meals. He was meticulous in his hygiene, and insisted that his appearance was of the utmost importance. Now the nurses caring for him notice that he is withdrawn and depressed. How can this patient and his relatives most effectively be supported through the various stages of their grief?

Situation 2

a) Mr. Thomas' confusion and inability to talk about his illness may result from denial of his condition. Our death is an inevitable prospect but it is not something that an individual usually focuses on; we usually dismiss it as an issue for old age. Mr. Thomas can only be helped by being allowed his denial.

b) Refusing to see his family, or in some cases, denying that they understand or care, results from the stage of anger. He fears that he is going to be forgotten. He mistrusts his family, his friends, staff, and other patients. The anger is deep and within himself. He demands attention and may be labelled by some staff as "a difficult patient". The nurses must at this stage do everything they can to allow him to express his anger; they must not judge his attention seeking as merely a way of getting what he wants.

c) The bargaining stage is shown by his meticulous hygiene, his demonstration that he has eaten his meals, and by waving to colleagues. He believes that bargaining is a way of controlling his fate. He feels that if he tries harder to do what he thinks is expected of him he will live longer. In a way, he is manipulating the situation much as a child manipulates his parents so that he may be in command.

d) In a way his depression goes hand in hand with the anger. Once anger is released the depression may be conquered. He may find it difficult to release his feelings by crying because of social attitudes. "Men don't cry" is a term we hear frequently. This is a stage that the patient has to deal with for himself, but not by himself.

e) Acceptance is a step towards attaining peace. Feelings are spent and conversation is unnecessary. When Mr. Thomas reaches such acceptance the nurses can show their caring by staying close and communicating in a non-verbal way in order to minimize the aloneness that he fears. It is now that his family will need the most support. Grief for them begins when they realize that their loss is inevitable. Mourning occurs over an extended period prior to death and will continue afterwards. Nurses need to recognise that relatives' behavioural changes, feelings of guilt, withdrawal of emotions, over-protection, and submissive courtesy, are indicators of their grief. Bereaved relatives may be supported through the early denial stage of their grief if they are encouraged or allowed to see the body; this will be painful, but it helps them to accept the fact of death. This is also the case when a child dies, or a baby is stillborn.

Conclusion

Bereavement can cause extreme unhappiness, but is an inevitable process in coming to terms with loss. It is essential that nurses give their whole support, love, and care to those in need and that they develop the counselling skills that are essential if we are to be able to give the best possible support. It should not be forgotten that counsellors themselves need support to continue to provide this care.

Reference

Kubler-Ross, E. (1969) On Death and Dying. Macmillan & Co, New York.

Bibliography

James, M., and Jongeward, D., (1978) Born to Win. American Library Inc., New York.
   An excellent book that contributes to our understanding of ourselves and others.

Nurse, G., (1980) Counselling and the Nurse. H.M. and M. Publishers Ltd., Aylesbury.
   This book gives a clear picture of counselling in use within nursing.

Rowan, J., (1983) The Reality Game. Routledge and Kegan Paul, London.
   A very useful book for anyone interested in psychotherapy.

Recent research shows that stigma attaches even to the most modern psychiatric service. As a professional you may give highly skilled help to patients with psychiatric problems, but how fully do you understand the problems of people who suffer social stigma as a result of seeking professional psychiatric help?

Managing psychiatric stigma

Kevin Teasdale, MA, Cert. Ed, RMN
Director of In-Service Training and Post Basic Nurse Education, Pilgrim Hospital, Boston, Lincs.

What is all the fuss about? "I think I would be too embarrassed to tell anyone I come to the day unit, because where we live they talk about the hospital as being a nuthouse and you hear people talking like that. So I'm frightened to let them know where I go. They think it's a lot of wild people running about."

That's how a client of a day unit described the stigma she felt from contact with the psychiatric service. A stigma is a discrediting and stereotyping label and the "madness" stigma is one of the most feared and damaging in our society. It is associated with loss of control, physical violence, and recovery is thought impossible. Many people think anyone who makes use of a psychiatric service is "mad".

The following situations could form the basis for discussion between you and your colleagues.

Situation 1 — How do patients manage stigma?
A patient about to be discharged from the psychiatric unit comes to you and says she is worried about how her friends and neighbours will treat her if she tells them where she has been. What is your opinion of the following strategies?
a) "I'm going to pretend I've been away visiting relatives."
b) "I'm going to tell them exactly where I've been and they can like it or lump it."
c) "It's all your fault for keeping me here. There never was anything wrong with me."
d) "I know they will never understand. This is the only place where people can accept me for what I am."

There is no single strategy for managing stigma so beware of giving advice. Help the patient to consider fully the advantages and disadvantages of each strategy to decide what is best for her.

a) Concealing a psychiatric history or "passing", as Goffman named it.

For: No one can stigmatise you if they cannot identify you as a former patient. Many people are so rigid in their views about mental illness that reasoning with them is a waste of time.

Against: You might be found out. Even if not, you will have to manage the stress of concealing the truth.

b) Being open.

For: It may be good for your self image. You could see yourself in a positive light if you come to terms with the stigma of contact with the psychiatric services. Degrees of open disclosure are possible. You may admit that you were in hospital but say that it was "only a nervous breakdown".

Against: Everyone in the neighbourhood will hear of your past, and some of them will avoid you, never giving you the chance to explain further.

c) Rejecting the Psychiatric Service — a form of selective disclosure.

For: It may be true and people will believe you. It may help to protect you from the trauma of wondering "Was I mad? Was I like those other patients?"

Against: People may not believe you. They will know that you were in hospital, and even worse will think you are still ill. You will be unable voluntarily to accept future psychiatric help, and may have to deny the value of any which has benefitted you in the past.

d) Rejecting the stigmatisers.

For: It may be true. In an area with a good hospital or social services network it may be quite possible to mix only with fellow patients and sympathetic carers.

Against: You will become isolated in the local community and very dependent on the caring services, which may be unable to meet all your needs.

Situation 2 — How aware are you?

Do you, perhaps unconsciously, react in a stereotyped and stigmatising way towards psychiatric patients. Have you ever:

a) Accepted praise for working with "people like that"?

b) Avoided patients when you see them in the street?

c) Pretended not to win when playing bingo with patients.

d) Sat with a group of staff at the back of the coach on a ward outing?

e) Dramatised violent incidents to entertain friends.

f) Joined in with a group of patients who are laughing at the antics of another disturbed patient?

g) Washed out a clean cup which patients sometimes use before drinking from it?

Depending on circumstances, any of these actions may be perfectly innocent or they may reveal a stigmatising attitude.

a) Innocent: The public is sympathetic to all nurses. The task of caring for dependent or disturbed patients is stressful and genuinely demanding.

Guilty: Many people are terrified of the very idea of mental illness and try to distance themselves from it. Anyone who volunteers to protect them from it by accepting praise reinforces the stereotype.

b) Innocent: The patient may not have wanted other people to know he had any contact with psychiatric services and you were being considerate. You were in a hurry and the patient is always talkative.

Guilty: You did not want to be seen talking to the patient in case other people thought you were a patient too. You like to keep private life separate from work — but would you still have this rule if you worked in an insurance office?

Find innocent and guilty explanations for the other examples. Remember that everyone who grew up in our society will have been exposed to the stereotypes of mental illness — the important thing is to become aware of them.

Situation 3 — What can you do to help?

A student nurse asks how he can help patients to manage the stigma of mental illness. What is your reaction to these suggestions.?

a) Encourage patients to discuss their fears about their own state of health and the reactions of others.

b) Make it clear that on the psychiatric unit a medical model is used. Patients who come here suffer from illnesses, are treated and usually make good recoveries.

c) Accept patients' own explanations about their illnesses — "I'm just depressed", even if you know that the doctor has diagnosed schizophrenia.

d) Organise a stigma management group to help patients learn from each other.

a) If a supportive approach is used, ventilation of thoughts and fears will help. Each patient must come to terms with how he interprets his own state of health as this will determine how he manages any stigma.

b) The philosophy of care — whether medical, social or any other — should be clear and consistent. Assess whether the model is acceptable to the patient. If necessary try to compromise.

c) There is no right or wrong answer to this one. A patient may try to deny the severity of his illness, and it would be unhelpful to reinforce this. But "depression" or "alcoholism" are likely to be more socially acceptable as explanations of psychiatric admission than "schizophrenia".

d) Stigma management lends itself well to group work. Help patients to share problems and strategies, and think out their implications. Give groups a sense of control by involving them in planning how the service can be presented to the public so as to reduce the stigma which attaches to it.

Situation 4 — What might happen in the group?

One patient in the stigma management group at a day unit reports that in applying for a part-time job, she has denied any psychiatric illnesses on the form she was sent. Another patient comments that this is dishonest. If you were the group leader would you use any of the following options, and how would you explain your choice?

a) Explain that she could be dismissed from the job later if the employers found out she had been lying.

b) Suggest that the group role-plays the job interview, exploring the different options of the interviewee and the possible reactions of the employer.

c) Agree with the second patient that honesty is the best policy.

d) Comment that for a part-time job you cannot see the relevance of detailed questions about medical history.

a) This is the present legal position. It might be useful to explain this to all the group members, on the basis that the more information they have, the better the basis on which they can make their decisions.

b) Role play is a very powerful way of exploring alternatives. It could be an elaborate rehearsal of the real interview situation, or brief question and answer discussion....?"

c) This goes against the principle of allowing group members to make up their own minds. In this example, the group leader is giving a personal opinion, whereas in a) he is stating facts. It could be argued that the leader of the group is entitled to give his own opinion. However, unless he himself has a psychiatric history, he will not have the same experience of being stigmatised as the other group members.

d) The same objections as in c) apply. The value of a well-run group is that group members learn from each other. The main reason for having an outsider as leader is to create an atmosphere of trust, and to ensure that personality clashes do not get in the way of calm exploration of options.

Conclusion

The advent of local psychiatric facilities may eventually help reduce the stigma of psychiatric care, but in the short term they make stigma management more difficult, because it is harder to conceal psychiatric contacts from the neighbourhood. Many patients feel very strongly about this, and are in great need of sensitive support and understanding from professionals.

Bibliography

Goffman, E. (1963) Stigma. Prentice Hall, New York. The basic work on the subject, written by a brilliant communicator.

Miles, A. (1984) The Stigma of Psychiatric Disorder: in Reed, J. and Lomas, G., Psychiatric Services in the Community, Croom Helm, London.

Meetings in psychiatric wards, attended by patients and staff, often appear to be disordered and full of trivia but they should not be taken at face-value. Closer examination reveals their administrative and clinical worth.

The psychiatric community meeting

Brendan McMahon, BA, SRN, RMN

Clinical Nurse Advisor in Psychotherapy, Southern Derbyshire Health Authority

Often the learner nurse's first experience of working in groups is the ward community meeting. This may be, or appear to be, a confused and confusing farrago of silence and anger, monologue and dialogue, sense and nonsense, interspersed with bizarre behaviour and frequent exits and entrances. What, one might think, is the point of all this? How can it possibly be conducive to patient health? In fact, psychiatric community meetings can have several useful functions.

Emotional and practical problems which are of concern to the whole ward community can be dealt with openly; these may include changes in ward structure, disruptive behaviour, departures and arrivals and similar issues which may arouse strong feeling. The ventilation of such feelings, which may be cathartic in itself, should also reduce the incidence of acting out in the ward, since, if frustrations can be shared they are less likely to result in physical aggression or self-destructive acts ('acting out' is a term for the expression of neurotic conflict in physical terms, eg hurting oneself or damaging property).

In any group of people living together in conditions which, often, do not allow much privacy, tensions develop. It is important to recognise and deal with them.

Supportive therapy can be carried out in community meetings, through sharing traumatic experience, family problems, and so on. There are advantages in having patients at different stages of their admission, as is usually the case on acute psychiatric wards. A patient who has come through a depressive episode, for example, may be in a unique position to inculcate hope in a patient who has just been admitted in the depths of depression and may believe that he will never feel any different. In such a situation, the sympathy and support of a fellow patient may be much more effective than that of the nurse.

Community meetings can be used to convey information in two directions:-

1. From the staff to patients. A common complaint of patients is that information is being kept from them. This is largely because of the hierarchical nature of communication on our wards. The consultant may come to some decision concerning an individual's treatment which will be communicated to the senior registrar, thence to the ward doctor who may then inform the senior nurse on duty, who may then delegate the task of telling the patient to a junior nurse. Somewhere along the line the message can become garbled or lost. Such patterns of communication can be altered, and by the constructive use of community meetings their worst effects can be obviated.

2. Communication 'upwards' from patients to staff can be encouraged, patients' views on their treatment can be elicited and taken into account in the formulation of treatment plans, and in this way patients can overcome their passivity and take an active part in their own recovery. 'Horizontal' communication between patients can also be enhanced.

Community meetings provide a unique opportunity for observing patient behaviour in inter-action with others, which may be very important diagnostically, in assessing need, and in the drawing-up of nursing care plans.

The meetings should not be used for reconstructure psychotherapy (that is, for the purpose of effecting fundamental changes in personality structure), since they lack the continuity and cohesiveness of small groups and are unselected, in that all members of the community are expected to attend.

Due to their primitive, unselected nature community meetings do present problems to the nurse therapist which she may not have encountered in other group settings. Among the most common are the following:

1. For some reason one patient refuses to attend a group meeting. This seems to strike a chord in the patients generally and some of the others ask why they should bother to attend. How should the nurse respond?

As a general point, it should be made clear to patients that attendance at community meetings is part of their treatment, and that it is therefore expected. It should also be remembered that no one should ever be coerced into attending any group.

Attendance invariably fluctuates according to the mood of the community, and people may not attend for a variety of reasons, including fear of confrontation, low morale, or unwillingness to share staff attention with others. In this particular case, the patient's refusal to attend should be traced to its underlying cause, expressed and resolved, as should the decision of other patients to collude with him. If community meetings are effectively conducted, a culture of attendance and participation can be nurtured. The level of attendance provides a useful indicator of morale on the ward.

2. There is a change in the atmosphere of the meeting. The patients in the group are uncommunicative and you suspect that the inhibiting factor is the presence of new unfamiliar student nurses at the ward meeting. How do you handle this situation?

On any given day, student, pupil or trained nurses, medical staff, social workers and social work students, occupational therapists and other members of staff on short, psychiatric placements may be present at a community meeting. Obviously this can have an inhibiting effect on patients and may arouse fantasies of being observed, studied and so on, especially if the newcomers, who often feel anxious themselves, sit silently throughout the meeting.

Patients should be encouraged to express any such underlying feelings, and helped to view them as understandable and acceptable. New students should be introduced and encouraged to say something about the reasons for their presence and expected length of stay. It is often useful for each member of the group to introduce himself to the newcomer by name; this may make the new staff member feel more at home and, so far as the patient group is concerned, help dispel paranoid fantasies and increase mutual awareness. If there are too many staff relative to patients, it may be advisable to limit staff attendance.

3. A patient who has been diagnosed as suffering from schizophrenia keeps bursting out laughing every time any group member says anything. As a consequence, communication is discouraged and the atmosphere is one of tense embarrassment. Should the nurse intervene and, if so, how?

When dealing with destructive or unsettled behaviour the principles involved are:
a. to help the group and the patient himself to understand what meaning is being communicated by such behaviour, that is, the reason why he is so anxious or angry;
b. to encourage him to develop more acceptable ways of expressing his feelings; and
c. to encourage the group to express its feelings about the behaviour and take some responsibility in helping the patient to control it.

The group will often look to the nurse to intervene directly, and occasionally this may be necessary for example by confronting the patient or insisting that he leaves. On the whole though, the nurse should encourage the meeting to deal with the problem in its own way: pressure from the patient's own peer group, that is, his fellow patients, will be more effective in modifying behaviour than any intervention the nurse might make.

4. One patient dominates the conversation, always bringing it back to his family problems. What are the options for handling this, and what are the principles involved?

The long, trivial discussions which often occur in community meetings are rarely so superficial as they appear. Frequently they indicate the presence of underlying preoccupations which are charged with anxiety, such as hostile feelings towards staff, fear of not getting better, fear of events moving out of control, and so on. These preoccupations may be expressed symbolically in the discussion of such topics as washing-up rotas, medication, or the quality of hospital food. In our present hypothetical case the nurse should use her understanding of the patient and of the group to look beneath his superficial chatter to the anxieties which lie below. If she is then able to encourage the patient to express those anxieties he can begin to resolve them and the troublesome behaviour will cease.

The chances of developing a cooperative, constructive community group culture are increased if meetings are held daily and at the same time. This is true of all types of groups in the ward setting. Their usefulness is enhanced if all ward staff emphasise the value of attendance.

Community meetings can be used for providing direct feedback of information from, for instance, ward rounds or care plan meetings, a much more economical use of time than conveying team decisions to patients on an individual basis. They can also be used for planning ward functions, parties, outings, and so on, since many patients have organisational or creative skills which remain untapped during their stay in hospital.

Utilising these skills reinforces self-esteem and the ability of individuals and the group to take decisions for themselves. Community meetings are of value in both clinical and management terms, and where such meetings do not take place, nurses would probably find it useful to ensure that they are set up as soon as is feasible.

Do our patients see what they need to see?
Are the caring team more concerned with a pleasant outlook than what is actualy visable within the immediate environment?
Often the "trivia" of everyday life is excluded from view while we blithely talk about the sunshine and flowers outside.

The patient's visual environment

Gillian B. Gough, SRN, SCM

Senior Sister, Ongoing Care Unit, The Churchill Hospital, Headington, Oxford

While the nursing team may be frustrated by the crumbling plaster and the need for new paint, the patient may be frustrated because he cannot get his hands on a newspaper or see a clock. Apparently, confused elderly people have been observed to undergo a change of personality, becoming outgoing and animated as soon as they know the time and have something to talk about.

Many elderly people lose touch with reality during their initial admission — they may be too apprehensive to hail the ward paperboy or venture to the hospital shop. Is it too much for us, as we rush about, to direct the paper seller to our patient? Do we remember to ask a relative to bring in an easily read clock if the ward clock is not visible — it may be inaccessible, too small or too high up to see. Our patients may be reluctant viewers of mundane sights, but how do we know what to obscure from view and what to leave? Screening the mortuary trolley may be appropriate in many areas where friends or relations feel it to be showing reverence and respect, but might some feel that this obscurity is a slight to the dead?

However, perhaps before considering final exits we should concentrate on arrival: it is reassuring and welcoming to see a smiling face; it is normal to see and wear our own clothes as we recover; it is lovely to see plants and flowers — especially those picked from home gardens or those of relatives; photographs of family, friends, and pets provide great comfort and assist those rehabilitating to reach their goals.

Pictures and photographs consolidate our patients' view of their life and achievements and are tangible evidence of their image and identity; they are often a source of pride for our patients and a major tool for their nurse. What about the ward photograph album? Photos of Christmas, day trips, patients' holidays — they all remind those in long-stay or high dependence situations that while their nursing care requirements may be very extensive, the world outside still exists and they are part of it — even if the ward windows are too high to view anything except the weather.

The outside world should be let in to be seen as well, for instance by colour television in a dayroom, personal television sets for those who like to view quietly in their own bedspace with their own choice of programmes. Free visiting usually results in a steady supply of new faces and visiting grandchildren (and even pets in some hospices) — all seen to be accessible as they would be at home, and they do much more psychological good than clinical harm, except of course, in acute clinical settings — walking, breathing manifestations of unclinical normality.

Calendars can be vital in any rehabilitation or ongoing care programme. In the absence of a personal calendar, a ward diary is a good substitute. They provide visible and tangible evidence that even if a certain goal is proving impossible to achieve, something is going to happen — we can see when an event important to our patient, which can be such an everyday matter as a hairdressing appointment, will take place and hopefully a certain amount of morale will stay intact.

The visual environment is also important for patients whose stay in hospital is only brief; for a newcomer to hospital (particularly a child) the unfamiliar environment can be bewildering and even frightening. Someone ill at home may suffer from the enforced restriction of the visual environment — a single room may become very monotonous. The visual environment perceived by someone who is partially sighted may be very different from that which others perceive. For someone who has experienced a change in their vision, their new experience of their environment is likely to be very frightening, and may shake their self-confidence, particularly when they try to walk around. Time should be made available to discuss their fears and new perceptions.

An "ideal" visual environment is rarely an inert and picturesque view, but rather one in which movement and variety help to reinforce a person's sense of normality.

The following situations and the discussion that accompanies them could be used as a starting point for thinking critically about the visual environment of *your* patients, or as the basis for discussion with colleagues.

Situation 1

Mrs Hicks, a long-stay patient, has developed a disconcerting habit of hiding food in a variety of places — it is often discovered in a mummified state on top of radiators or beneath the rather high ward windows, and one day she is even seen hurling her sandwiches at the window panes.

After the incident of the thrown sandwiches, Mrs Hicks finally confides that she has been trying to feed the birds and has been storing food for them. The solution in this case was the provision of a bird-table outside the much lower dayroom window. Mrs Hicks always makes a bee-line for a chair near this window anyway, and from that point on the discovery of her little stocks diminished and feeding the birds became a routine controlled by Mrs Hicks.

Situation 2

Jeremy has recently been moved onto the children's ward where the only bed available was in a corner. He is very miserable and at night spends a lot of time lying on his back staring at the ceiling. He does not sleep well and does not talk much.

When the library trolley came round, the librarian suggested that Jeremy couldn't lie on his left-hand side because of his operation, and lying on his other side meant that all he could see was the blank wall. He then said that he had never been able to sleep on his back and didn't like sleeping facing the wall because it was "too black at night". The solution was supplied by another child on the ward who volunteered to change beds since she was partially sighted and would be happier and feel more secure in a corner bed where she could orientate herself better. Both children had been too scared of "causing a fuss" to complain before.

Situation 3

Mr Bell is a recently admitted dysphasic patient, whose refusal of morning medication is rapidly becoming routine. His routine does, however, include a newspaper which he reads while having his breakfast. After a while it was observed that on many occasions Mr Bell would take his medication if his nurse took the time to flick through the pages briefly, discussing and commenting on news items.

While Mr Bell's vision enabled him to read the items himself, he needed to share what he saw in order to grasp the reality of it from the very different world he was inhabiting on the ward. Exchange of views and discussion with his nurse meant that she was also participating in this normal breakfast time event. The situation clarified and routine adjusted, Mr Bell usually took his tablets.

Situation 4

Six-year old Susan has come into hospital for the first time and clearly feels very threatened by her new environment. She explains to a staff nurse that "everything seems so big".

The staff nurse encourages Susan to describe what she can see: the other beds, the trolleys, the big double-doors and so on, and to make up stories about them, so that they become more familiar to her. The staff nurse also asks Susan's mother to bring in a few more of Susan's own toys, so that she has more of her own things around her.

Situation 5

Miss Daisy Brown has spent a lifetime in institutional care. At the age of 90 she participated in the ward holiday and went to the coast for the first time in her life. She enjoyed herself immensely, having experienced many new things for the first time, and joined in enthusiastically with all the activities that she could. Her sight is failing, and since her return she is erratic in her mood, often crying because she had to come back.

The nurses rapidly processed the photographs and purchased some large picture frames (easily felt as well as seen). Certificates (she won many prizes on the holiday — her extrovert character ensured that) and pictures were displayed around her bed and in the dayroom and her prizes viewed and discussed. Miss Brown became much happier; the evidence of her success and experience were there for all to share and admire and she was able to keep the memory of her enjoyment much fresher and feel that it was still with her.

Situation 6

Michael Summers returned home a week ago with extensive plaster casts resulting from multiple fractures he had received in an accident at work. He is immobile, and will be for several weeks, and is already finding the bedroom he is in very boring. The tantalizing glimpses of the garden seem to make the frustration even worse.

The solution was found by his children, who painted huge posters with widely differing scenes on them, which they hung on the bedroom walls, replacing them with new ones as often as they could. His daughter drew some cut-out characters which could be moved around the posters every time someone came into the room.

Situation 7

Mrs Moor frequently complains of blurred vision — her symptoms and severity of problem vary from hour to hour. Specialist referrals have yielded little result. We observe her problems to be worse after meals.

The solution is very simple. This lady is very active, taking her glasses on and off, putting them down in all sorts of places and most of all fingering the lens when she has eaten something sticky. The remedy lies in cleaning her glasses after every meal and more frequently if necessary. Her field of vision is then clear and Mrs Moor is content.

In the problems discussed it is interesting that often what is seen needs to be shared; not only must things be seen and done, they must also be talked about. Sound and vision are partners, and perhaps as well as worrying about what we see on our wards we need to concentrate on what we can say about it. Try, also, to imagine how the ward appears to an outsider. When you spend a lot of time in a particular environment it can become difficult to "see" it properly, and a fresh mind and eye can often suggest improvements and solutions to problems and annoyances that your patients have just put up with, either because they don't like to cause a fuss or because they can't express their frustration.

Bibliography

(1974) Notes on Nursing (Chapter IX Light) Florence Nightingale Blackie, Glasgow and London
Remains relevant to all aspects of modern nursing — her empathy with the patient is very apparent. The most perceptive thing I have read on this topic.

Noise! Does it soothe or alarm? How can we ensure the sounds our patients hear have a positive rather than a negative effect upon their recovery and quality of life?

The patient's auditory environment

Gillian Gough, SRN, SCM

Senior Sister, Ongoing Care Unit, The Churchill Hospital, Headington, Oxford

Stress results from unwanted noise. This applies as much to our homes, the street, or place of work, as it does to our patients and stress is recognised as the cause of a myriad of problems from inhibited wound healing to behavioural problems (both in patients and staff).

Acceptable noise levels mean different things to different people. The music blasting from the ward radio resulting from the domestic needing something to raise her spirits and energy levels is just an excrutiating racket to the aphasic patients unable to tell her what they think of it. What about the chairbound person in the dayroom who may fall victim to the ambulant, determined character mesmerised by the volume control on the television, or the comatose patient whose relatives insist on discussing him loudly at the bedside oblivious to the fact that our first sense to develop is the last to leave us, or the inexperienced or insensitive team member who exhibits the same behaviour when "caring" for the unresponsive or those considered to be out of earshot.

Communication between staff that results in misunderstanding and leads to ineffective care is obviously as harmful to the recipient as the carer who doesn't take the time to ensure her partially hearing or deaf patient understands what is being said and what is going on.

The lady who suddenly exhibits paranoid tendencies may have overheard the television or radio and whilst in a sedated or partially hearing state has totally misunderstood her environment. She in turn may start a chain reaction, becoming frightened and noisy — in turn alarming other patients with the same results. This is particularly relevant to wards caring for the elderly whose total awareness is reduced by multiple sensory impairments.

Lack of noise may be equally upsetting, as may individual changes in a person's own hearing. Noise in its absence or excess is often a larger problem than we realise. I will not dwell on raised voices, squeaking equipment, banging doors and trolleys — they speak for themselves too often.

The following situations and suggested remedies could be used as a starting point for thinking critically about your patients' auditory environment or as the basis for discussion with colleagues.

Situation 1

Miss Green aged 80, is overheard muttering about being arrested and refusing to wear her brooch because she is on probation. This is not the first time she has exhibited this behaviour.

a) Should we tell her that she is imagining things?

b) How can we reduce her anxiety?

c) Are factors other than auditory contributing to her problems?

a) Ask her why she feels these things are happening. In this case it was found that she had overheard the television in the adjacent dayroom. The caring team must also exclude urinary tract infection resulting in urinary retention, constipation, dehydration and reactions to drugs or hallucinations resulting from over-sedation as a cause. Ear syringing and the provision of a hearing aid may also be found to be indicated if her hearing is impaired.

b) By providing a bed away from the dayroom and ensuring that when she chooses to enter this area she knows the television is on and her hearing aid is functioning properly, the risk of misperception is reduced. The nursing staff should also provide the necessary support in the form of clear unhurried speech and reassuring physical contact.

c) The problems presented in (a) may be exacerbated by partial or total loss of vision making discrimination and the tendency to misunderstand more frequent. The television or radio can be used positively to reinforce reality, news items, time and weather checks can give proper dimensions to time and location to those without sight.

Situation 2

Mr Smith is a dysphasic gentleman in a long stay environment, he is prone to making violent gestures and bellowing at the top of his voice — often throughout the night. He is hemiplegic and suffers the occasional bout of urinary incontinence.

a) Are the problems greatest for Mr Smith, the other patients or the ward staff?
b) Why does he do it?
c) Can he stop it? Should we intervene?

a) The problems affect each group. Mr Smith's distress is obvious, the other patients are disturbed, the nursing staff must act in a situation with a rapidly increasing level of stress.

b) Frustration and his inability to express a need are the usual cause.

c) Yes he can, a checklist of "wants" usually produce a result, soothing music may also help him (and others). However, simple exuberance and the need to express his feelings can produce a "melodious blast". It would be inappropriate to curb this as happiness is hopefully infectious.

Situation 3

Emma Sampson is seven years old and lives with her parents and four very lively brothers in a small house on the other side of town. She has just been admitted to the isolation ward, in a room on her own, with suspected typhoid, following a family holiday in Morocco. She has a temperature of 40.5°C (105°F), and is suffering from diarrhoea and vomitting. Her mother is visiting her every day. She is hardly sleeping at all and complains frequently that "hospital is a very creepy place".

When Staff Nurse Susan Morgan asks her what she means, it becomes clear that she is upset by the silence and loneliness of the isolation unit and by the fact that everyone is wearing masks, gloves and gowns. What would help Emma to feel more at ease?

Emma is used to a boisterous and noisy, busy environment at home (and probably at school, too). A radio or cassette player with her favourite music may help to counteract the silence of her environment, and this and some of her toys and pictures may help to make her feel more at home. Her illness and the unfamiliar environment will enhance her feelings of isolation. Her mother or father could be encouraged to come in and stay with her; this would reduce her sense of isolation and be very comforting for her.

Nurses need not use masks and gowns when caring for Emma, as long as they are aware of the likely routes of spread of the suspected disease and use meticulous hygiene when handling her blood or faeces. Emma's sense of isolation amounts to much more than just the deprived auditory environment.

Situation 4

Mrs Mills is an active lady, thriving in an ongoing care situation. She is apparently deaf and is referred to the ENT Department where she creates havoc. One day she finally returns with a hearing aid and an embarrassed escort. Within three days the hearing aid has vanished, rumour has it that it has been "flushed down the toilet" amidst declarations of "I'm not deaf so there!" Questioning results in requests to speak in "this ear please, I can't hear you".

a) What are the benefits of being deaf?
b) What is alarming about a brand new hearing aid?
c) Can we resolve the situation and would it be appropriate?

a) An excuse to ignore people and requests that meet with disapproval. It is also a foolproof method for close contact as the speaker offers an arm and talks into your ear — this can be a prime motive.

b) Suddenly being able to hear may be intolerable, apart from volume of sound, background noise previously unheard may be irritating.

c) In many cases extra attention may be the answer. However some patients use deafness as a way of maintaining control on their own terms. This is an integral part of their personalities and in such cases a hearing aid is inappropriate.

Situation 5

John Daniels has just undergone neuro-surgery to remove a large meningioma and is making an uneventful recovery in the intensive care unit. His only complaint is that everyone seems to be speaking with very high-pitched voices. What is the most helpful nursing response to this?

The presence of the tumour, increasing in volume gradually, has imposed considerable pressure on the neighbouring region of the brain, including the auditory cortex. The functioning of this has adapted gradually with the increasing pressure, which has been released with the removal of the tumour. This has given John Daniels a distorted perception of sound, which will gradually re-adapt to normal functioning over a period of days. He would benefit from a careful explanation of the situation and the expected recovery. He may also experience balance and visual problems for similar reasons and could be warned about these. Various drugs, including some antibiotics can affect the patient's perceived hearing; with prolonged use, or high dosages some of these changes may be irreversible.

Conclusion

As these examples show, the auditory environment is only one part of the patient's *sensory* environment, and hearing is often inextricably linked with the information about the environment available from the other senses. The patient's *complete* environment therefore needs careful consideration.

Bibliography

Nightingale, F. (1974) Notes on nursing. Blackie and Son Ltd, Glasgow and London. Chapter IV (Noise).

Wells, T.J. (1980) Problems in geriatric care. Churchill Livingstone, Edinburgh, London and New York. Chapter 8.

How do those charged with investigating a disputed incident get to the truth? The evidence must be carefully examined and those involved must be asked the right questions. This Practice Check suggests some ways of sharpening up investigations.

Questioning skills: investigating a disputed incident

David Carson, LLB

Senior Lecturer, Faculty of Law, University of Southampton

How do you ask questions? There is a skill in interviewing people for a job or counselling colleagues, but is there also one in asking questions when investigating a disputed incident? You could be investigating a patient's complaint, considering an allegation of professional misconduct, deciding whether an injury to a child was non-accidental, finding out how an accident took place. How do you get useful, accurate information? Do you sometimes feel like a police officer or lawyer but lack their training or experience?

This article outlines some ways of asking questions when there is a dispute about what happened. It will not produce easy answers where none are available but it will certainly help to get answers where they are available. It is based on a number of workshops and role-plays where nurses and others investigated a mock incident. Two contrasting styles of questioning stood out at those workshops. Most nurses seemed to collect as much information about an incident as was possible before they reflected on it and reached their decision. They also paid a lot of attention to feelings, motivation and relationships. It is suggested that this approach is not as effective as the alternative, in which answers are critically assessed as soon as they are given. On receiving an answer, the questioner considers whether it can be checked or made more or less believable. Also, in this approach, feelings and motivations are treated as facts to be questioned and assessed like all the other evidence.

It would be wrong to consider this second approach as hostile or designed to frighten the people being questioned. That is certainly not intended and is likely to be counterproductive. It need not involve disbelieving or distrusting the person but trying to make as strong a case as possible. However, there is a danger in that the procedure can be made so obvious that a dishonest person could use it to make a strong false case. It must be used sensibly and subtly.

Mental role-plays

When investigating a factual dispute, use the information you are given to create a 'mental picture' of the scene and people involved. As the action is described it will become a 'mental role-play'. The questioner is told who did what, when, where and how. This must be fitted into the picture. Any pieces that do not fit — he was in the doorway when he grabbed the knife — suggest further questions to explain the difficulties or isolate the discrepancy. It should be done slowly, quietly and indirectly. The essential feature is seeking information to confirm or deny the information already given.

- Spend some time 'in the shoes' of the different people involved in the incident. Go through the motions that have been described to 'see' if they are possible or likely. Could I have moved from there to here in that time?
- Think about what you would have done. If that had happened to me would I have done that and, if not, is it believable that he or she did?
- Think about what would be visible and audible to whom. Was it?
- Think about the traces. What signs or physical evidence like injuries or broken property are there? This is always useful evidence.
- Think about the evidence that is *not* there. If it had happened in that way what would you expect to have happened, been seen, heard, felt, smelt, tasted? Which traces, for example skid marks or broken banisters, would you expect to exist? Do they? If not, why not?
- Think about reflex actions. Did the person do what he or she normally would, for example use the same language, when there was no opportunity to think about doing something different.
- Think about normal practices and procedures. We usually do the same thing in the same way, we are creatures of habit, so if this act was unusual, why?
- Think about the causal chain. Do the causes or events link together fully and credibly?
- Think about additional and alternative theories and explanations. Did or could something else have caused it or contributed to it happening that way? We often emphasise or concentrate on one cause or factor when others deserve examination.

Having collected, and critically assessed the evidence it will often be wise to act out the incident, if possible in the place where it occurred. Does the oral description match the re-enactment? Does the re-enactment contradict the answers given earlier? The oral information must have been collected in full before any re-enactment takes place or the witnesses could learn from it how to describe what happened.

Yes, 'mental role-plays' could help the liar. But few people will have the time, ability, or opportunity, particularly if investigations are prompt, to think through all the details. Remember, they would have to think through something that did not happen which is much harder to role-play.

This approach can also be used where it is the motivation for rather than the behaviour that is disputed. A nurse says she was rude to a patient because she was in a rush to keep an appointment with the ward sister. Mentally role-play it.

Would you be rude in such circumstances? Would you not prefer sister's praise for putting the patient first? Is the nurse's answer consistent with the claimed motivation?

Professional misconduct

You are the sister or charge nurse of a general medical ward. On returning to the ward after a meeting, a patient, Mrs Colby, tells you that Nurse Archer slapped her across the face. Her right cheek looks a little pink. Mrs Colby explains that Nurse Archer has never liked her. Nurse Archer was reluctant to do things for her like bring a cup of coffee to the bed. Indeed when she had eventually done so, that afternoon, Nurse Archer had taken the opportunity to slap Mrs Colby while she was holding her cup of coffee.

You have heard nothing about a poor relationship between Nurse Archer and Mrs Colby. She is in a low dependency, six-bedded cubicle and due for discharge in two days time. There are three other patients in that ward.

Nurse Archer has finished her shift and gone home but Nurse Dale recalls helping Nurse Archer — who had seemed a little upset — change Mrs Colby's bed and wipe up some coffee and a broken saucer from the floor by the bed. When you question Nurse Archer the next morning she is anxious, hostile and suspicious. She accuses you of believing patients before colleagues.

Decide what questions you are going to ask. Create a mental picture of the ward and role-play the actions as best you can. Think of the kind of information that could help you and test the different theories about what might have happened. Go through the list of ideas above. You may be on the right track, but until we have interactive journals, I cannot tell. Consider whether your questions would seek the following useful information. It is just a selection to illustrate this technique. Many more questions could be asked and ideas followed up.

Is Nurse Archer left or right-handed? Which side of the bed did she approach? If she came to Mrs Colby's right-hand side and is right-handed then it is unlikely that she would have slapped Mrs Colby's right cheek, which is what you were told. Where was the coffee spilt? If it went over the centre of the bed, this suggests it was pushed at the patient. But if it went on the floor and the right-hand side of the bed this suggests it was pushed at the nurse by the patient. You were told there were traces of coffee on the floor and that a saucer broke. Independent corroboration is available from Nurse Dale. When did it happen? Should any slap marks have disappeared by the time Sister saw Mrs Colby? Where were the other patients? Could they have seen and heard? Was Nurse Archer in the way? What was heard and in what order? Would you exclaim if coffee was spilt on you? Who did? Was that before or after the slap, if any? What normally happens when a nurse does not 'get on' with a patient? Did it, and if not, why not?

This imaginary case is also used in a 30 minute video-programme, produced for and available from Wessex RHA, entitled "Witnessing in Disciplinary Appeals." It demonstrates the kind of trouble a ward sister could get into, during disciplinary proceedings, when questioned by a skilled representative determined to show how poorly the case was investigated. It also shows how it should have been done.

Fell or pushed?

Bobby Ewing, aged 6, is brought to casualty, shoeless and in pyjamas, with severe bruises to his torso and limbs. His mother, Pam, explains: "I'd overslept. My husband had already left for work. We were going to be late for school. I went in and woke Bobby. As usual he didn't want to stir or shower. I told him to get washed and dressed and I went downstairs to prepare breakfast. A few minutes later I heard a long series of bumps and Bobby screaming. I found him in an awkward twisted position right at the bottom of the stairs. I also spotted one of his favourite toy cars near him. He must have been playing with it, put it down, stood on it and slipped all the way down the stairs. I immediately picked him up and put him in the car. No, he didn't lose consciousness, vomit or complain of double vision, and no, I cannot explain why he says I pushed him down the stairs unless it is to punish me for making him get up."

Again, what kind of information would you like to have to help you decide whether Mrs Ewing is lying. Once you know what information you want you can formulate your question.

You should find out what the house and stairs look like. If the stairs have a turn in them then it is unlikely that Bobby could have fallen from top to bottom. Where was the toy usually kept? If not tidied away how did the adults miss slipping on it the night before and in the morning? If they were in his bedroom how did they come out? Why did he play on the landing — it could be colder than in his bedroom? Would the landing have more attractions? He was reluctant to get up. If that is so, and he started off by playing with his toys, is five minutes realistic? The toy went down the stairs. That suggests he would slip with his feet going forwards and wouldn't most of the injuries be to his back? If he had had his back to the stairs when he slipped, head first, the toy would have stayed upstairs. Would he have any cause, particularly as still in his pyjamas, to walk towards, as opposed to past, the top of the stairs? In other words if he slipped on a toy wouldn't he normally fall sideways along the landing? Was Mrs Ewing dressed before she went into his room? No. Then did she dress before taking him to casualty, which indicates a lack of care? Yes. Then wouldn't you wake up the others, before getting dressed yourself, because it saves time and allows closer supervision? Test the motivation as well as the facts.

These techniques will not provide the answer; they are only offered as a way of sharpening up investigations and questions.

Questions about the actors' relationships with and feelings towards each other are still relevant. This paper will have succeeded if it encourages more questions about and assessments of the likelihood of the facts being as they are told.

Aggression on the ward, on the part of patients or staff, can be very disruptive. How do you cope with its occurrence on your ward? This Practice Check can be used to start discussion of how to handle it.

Handling aggression

Ruth E. Smith, BSc, RGN, RMN, DN Cert
Support Worker in Rehabilitation, Lothian Regional Council, Department of Social Work

Aggression may occur in many situations, and may be healthy or unhealthy. It may be caused by a number of factors, and may occur in a variety of social environments, including all the possible settings for care. Your response will influence the outcome, and may:
● Minimise the potential for aggressive or violent behaviour.
● Reduce the likelihood of its recurrence.
● Provoke the onset of aggressive or violent behaviour.
● Offer opportunities for further attacks by the aggressor.
Carefully read the situations described below and select the response, or responses, you consider to be most appropriate. Remember that there are few "right" or "wrong" answers, but certain responses are more likely to minimise or eliminate the potential for aggressive or violent behaviour.

The following situations could form the basis for discussion between yourself and colleagues

1. You are asked to talk to a group of student nurses whose main worry is the fear of violence. How would you approach this:
   a) Give a lecture on the theories of aggression?
   b) Give a lecture on the practicalities of handling an aggressive outburst?
   c) Use research to show that their fears are not justified?
   d) Use a video illustrating aspects of violence?
   e) Use role play or close-circuit television to provide feedback on the students' own skills in handling violence?

The approach in teaching students should allow them to discuss their fear and gain confidence in handling an aggressive outburst.
   Start with a short talk on the theories of aggression · outline precipitating factors, particularly those under the nurses' control; talk should include recent research. Give out a factsheet on the practicalities of dealing with an aggressive outburst. Explore the students' fears. Use role play or video or both, to illustrate an incident. Allow students sufficient time to absorb information given: this may take a whole day, during which library time for private study could be included to form a break from the classroom. The students' own experience of past aggressive behaviour while caring could usefully be discussed and explored.

a) *For:* Emphasising that aggression is part of us all is worthwhile, and identifying factors that predispose individuals to behave aggressively is very important.
Against: This will not necessarily reduce the students' own fears, since it relies heavily on the students' level of participation and involvement in the discussion.
b) *For:* This information is closer to what the students want.
Against: Giving the information in a lecture form may make it seem far removed from the ward situation. A handout for future reference may be more useful, although very few written guidelines can be sufficiently comprehensive to be really useful.
c) *For:* Research is important in any teaching session.
Against: Unless supplemented by other teaching, the students may feel that their fears are seen as "stupid".
d) *For:* These can be "stopped" or "played back" — time must be allowed for the students to comment on action the nurse could or should have taken.
Against: Students may themselves "switch off". There are very few video films of suitable depth and quality available.
e) *For:* This is a beneficial way of learning — it allows students to confront the feared situation and receive direct feedback. You need to allow time for discussion. Verbal and non-verbal responses can be illustrated.
Against: It demands a certain degree of willingness and confidence on the part of the students. Good audio visual facilities are needed for close-circuit TV.

2. You are a ward sister or charge nurse and you arrive · on the ward to discover two of the nurses in tears after being verbally abused by a patient who is clearly in a very emotional state. Who would you speak to first:
   a) The patient?
   b) The nurses who are upset?
   c) The nurse in charge of the ward?
   d) The medical staff?
   e) The clinical nurse manager?

a) *For:* The patient is obviously distressed — he may be verbally abusive to another member of staff or patient, he may resort to physical violence. You need to establish what led the patient to abuse the nurses.
Against: Unless you have a good relationship with the patient you may increase the likelihood of a further outburst. Without spending a long time with the patient it is unlikely that a clear understanding of the incident will be gained.
b) *For:* The nurses will feel that they have support from a senior member of staff. You need to ascertain the sequence of events that led to the outburst.
Against: This will not ease the tension among the other

The ideal response should aim to prevent any further abuse and to reduce both the patient's and the nurses' distress. Discover as quickly as possible the circumstances — assess the risk of future abuse (verbal or physical) and the number of staff available. A senior member of staff who knows the patient should discuss the incident with him or be in his immediate vicinity. If there is a probability of future abuse, medical staff and nurse managers should be informed immediately. A senior member of staff should take the nurses who are upset away from the situation and allow them to discuss the incident. As many staff as possible should remain on the ward, to support both each other and the other patients. The incident should be discussed fully with all the ward team — the aim being to prevent a recurrence.

staff or patients, and you may not get an accurate account of what occurred.

c) *For:* You should be able to ascertain the circumstances surrounding the outburst and assess the risk to other staff and patients.
Against: The situation may escalate when senior members of staff are not in the vicinity.

d) *For:* This may provide more information and ward staff on the ward.
Against: It may take time that could be better used in directly defusing the situation.

e) **As d).** As ward manager you can support the situation by deploying staff from another area to help until calm returns to the ward. A situation of this sort should always be reported to the clinical nurse manager.

---

3. You are a ward sister or charge nurse and the attitude of a senior student nurse is causing you concern. She appears to be inflexible in her approach and abrasive in manner. This has resulted in a shouting match beween her and a patient, who was previously calm and undemanding. Would you:
   a) Report the nurse to the nurse manager, or to the students' tutor or DNE, or both?
   b) Talk with the patient?
   c) Send the nurse off the ward, perhaps back to the college or school of nursing to see a tutor there?
   d) Talk with the nurse?

The ideal response should aim to encourage the nurse to explore her attitude and to identify the reasons why she provokes aggressive responses from patients. Allow the nurse to present her view of the situation, particularly her feelings. Focus on the nurse's responses. What caused her to respond in that way? Could she have responded differently? Encourage her to question her own attitude. If she appears unable or unwilling to do this then you may have to confront her, and if necessary report the situation. Next time act sooner.

a) *For:* They may give you more support should further action need to be taken. The patient may complain in writing to the Health Authority about this incident, and a written report is recommended.
Against: It would not change the present situation or help the student nurse.

b) *For:* The patient is obviously angry and distressed and needs to discuss what has happened. The patient needs reassuring that the behaviour of the nurse will not be repeated.
Against: It does not appear to be the patient's attitude that provoked the outburst.

c) *For:* This would temporarily relieve the tension on the ward.
Against: The situation may recur because nothing is being resolved.

d) *For:* It will establish whether it is the nurse's attitude that appears to be the problem.
Against: Unless carefully handled, the nurse may feel that she has been wronged.

---

4. You are a ward sister or charge nurse and a patient who assaulted two nurses during his last admission is being re-admitted. How do you prepare the nursing team:
   a) Say nothing?
   b) Ask for extra nursing staff?
   c) Arrange a senior staff meeting to discuss the patient?
   d) Arrange a teaching session for nursing staff?

The ideal response should aim to ensure the highest standard of care for the patient with the minimum risk to staff. Involve all levels of nursing staff. Examine the circumstances surrounding the last admission, in particular the violent behaviour. If the minutes from the last post-incident meeting are available these should be read and discussed. Have the circumstances changed? What can be learned from past behaviour? Could nursing staff have prevented the behaviour? How can risk be minimised? Ensure staff know hospital policy – basic guidelines on how to respond, such as how to get the extra help. Further sessions during patient's stay should monitor the situation, including the level of staff stress.

a) *For:* This will prevent the patient's reputation influencing nurses' behaviour, provided that none of your team have met him before.
Against: It is unethical to withhold relevant information and may put staff at greater risk.

b) *For:* This will ensure a greater number of staff are available should violent behaviour seem likely.
Against: It may increase staff and other patients' anxieties regarding the patient in question.

c) *For:* This will ensure senior staff are aware of the situation. A plan of action to reduce the potential for his aggressive behaviour should be drawn up, providing each member of staff with direction on what to do, and when, why, and how to take action.
Against: Junior staff, including nursing students, may feel more threatened if they feel that they lack support. It may therefore be advisable to include them in these discussions.

d) *For:* This allows not only the situation but also ways of coping with it to be explored.
Against: It may be difficult for all staff to attend.

Bibliography

Atkinson, R., Atkinson R., and Hilgrad, E., (1983) Introduction to Psychology, 8th edition. Harcourt, Brace, and Jovanovich, New York.
A good reference book covering all areas of psychology.

Glynn Owens, R., and Barrie Ashcroft J., (1985) Violence — A Guide for the Caring Professions, Croom Helm Ltd.
Views the problem of violence from three different perspectives (biological, social and psychological) and includes research findings. Detailed reading in the study of violence.

Morris, D., (1979) Manwatching. Jonathan Cape Ltd., London.
Enjoyable reading which will tell you a lot, not only about others' behaviour but also your own.

Royal College of Psychiatrists and Royal College of Nursing (1985) The Principles of Good Medical and Nursing Practice in the Management of Violence in Hospital. RCN London.
Practical suggestions for nursing/hospital policy and 'on the ward' situations. May be available in Nursing/Medical Libraries.

Storr, A., (1968) Human Aggression, Pelican Books, England.
Worth reading for an overall view of aggression.

Caring for people is a stressful occupation. Compound this with the everyday problems of inadequate staffing levels, low pay, unfamiliar procedures, overtime, and patients' deaths, and nurses can become victims of burnout. Could you recognise the signs, and would you know what action to take?

Can you recognise burnout?

Elizabeth M. Horne, MA
Editorial Director, The Professional Nurse

Burnout is more than the state of physical, emotional, and mental exhaustion which may accompany stress. It is a condition in which, at worst, its sufferer experiences chronic fatigue and a total loss of purpose and enthusiasm due to complete dissipation of energy. The symptoms provoked by stress should be distinguished from those of burnout, which is a much more serious condition and may result from a situation of continuing or increasing stress (Table 1).

A certain level of stress is an essential ingredient for effective and innovative working and living, and people respond differently to this stimulus. Those who are most highly motivated, committed, and enthusiastic, and who have apparently limitless energy and a tendency toward perfectionism, can be among the most innovative and inspiring people in a department; their activity and enthusiasm is often a major asset.

However, these are the very people most at risk from burnout, especially where they are striving for high standards in an inflexible system with inadequate resources and working increasing amounts of overtime to the exclusion of friends and recreation.

Those nurses who are under stress may risk developing burnout and they have a responsibility, towards their colleagues and themselves, to recognise the process if it begins to occur (Cherniss, 1980).

The burnout process is a continuous one, but four stages can be identified (Edelwich and Brodsky, 1980).

Enthusiasm: This is an essential quality for all nurses, and many people enter the profession, or start a new job, with great energy, commitment, high ideals, and a determination to provide the best care for their patients. They are willing to take on extra work, often to compensate for inadequate resources, to ensure that a high quality of patient care is maintained. Nursing is by its nature stressful, and if the everyday stresses are combined with an increasing workload inevitably some parts of the nurse's work no longer match up to her ideals.

Stagnation: The individual's enthusiasm and motivation are dulled as expectations are thwarted.

Frustration: The previously well-motivated professional becomes frustrated and cynical as she realises that she cannot change the system and achieve her ideals. Her emotional reserves are depleted, and she experiences a sense of personal failure.

Withdrawal: A form of depression follows in which the ability to cope is lost; decision making, even on minor matters, is difficult and causes anxious uncertainty; work breaks may become long and the individual becomes isolated. This state of chronic collapse can be termed "burnout".

At an early stage during this process, the intervention (either by the individual herself, or by a colleague or peer) of realistic goals and expectations, and the regular opportunity to cut off from work and replenish resources, can reverse the process. The further the condition has developed, the longer recovery takes.

If the value of an individual's work and achievements is positively acknowledged by colleagues and peers, and trust exists between members of the caring team so that a high level of communication occurs, the risk of burnout is dramatically reduced. Effective management to create such a team is an essential defence against burnout, and can encourage personal growth and support within the group.

Table 1. Symptoms provoked by stress and burnout (Adapted from Niehouse, 1981)

Stress	Burnout
Fatigue	Chronic exhaustion
Anxiety	Unfulfilled need for recognition
Dissatisfaction	Boredom or cynicism
Less commitment	Detachment/denial of feelings
Moodiness	Impatience or irritability
Guilt	Depression
Poor concentration	Disorientation/forgetfulness
Physiological changes	Psychosomatic complaints

The following situations could form the basis for discussion between yourself and colleagues.

1. Which are most likely to help a colleague minimise stress and avoid developing burnout?
   a) Occasional (and honest) praise for their work.
   b) A cut in staffing levels in their department.
   c) Regular "social" conversation with colleagues on topics unrelated to work.
   d) The opportunity to talk openly, in confidence, about their feelings.
   e) An additional new and challenging responsibility.

Situation 1
a, c and **d** are the most helpful in preventing burnout; they maintain a sense of purpose and achievement and prevent a sense of isolation. A new challenge (**e**) can re-awaken some enthusiasm, but may also present an additional burden.

2. Which of the following suggest that you may risk developing burnout?
   a) You start categorising your patients as symptoms rather than people.
   b) You find yourself concentrating exclusively on only one part of your job.
   c) You frequently socialise with your colleagues.
   d) The number of occasions on which you work long hours of overtime is increasing.
   e) You feel a professional distance between yourself and your patients.

Situation 2
a, b and **d.** Losing a personal human interest in your patients; concentrating only on one part of your job; and working long hours of overtime are symptoms of stress which could develop into burnout.

3. Which of the following nurses is at most risk of developing burnout?
   a) Susan Alexander is a highly motivated and very competent staff nurse who has just moved from a small rural hospital to a large city general hospital. She is horrified to find her ward is understaffed and that the cleaners have been working to rule for five months. Morale is low and patient care, by her high standards, is barely adequate. She hasn't yet had time to get to know anyone in the area and is too tired to go out and meet people. She feels able to talk about her feelings only with the night-duty sister, who is about to leave.
   b) Bill Johnson, a charge nurse for five years in a busy male surgical ward, has uncompromisingly high standards in running the ward. He has just joined a rock band, as lead guitarist. He is now spending more time and energy practising his guitar and is beginning to juggle his duty hours to accommodate band practice and concert times.
   c) Sheila North is a third-year student nurse who clearly feels a sense of great commitment to her patients. She makes great efforts to get to know each of them personally, and is always willing to listen to their problems. Patients and colleagues alike appreciate her kind and caring approach and tell her so. She is beginning to work overtime to give patients extra support, and even to keep in touch with them once they've returned home. Her only other pre-occupation seems to be the work she's doing in preparation for her finals.

Situation 3
a: Susan's approach may put her at great risk from developing burnout, especially once the only colleague she confides in has moved away. If she can readjust her expectations to a more realistic level, and allow herself more time and energy to develop activities and friends outside work, she may be able to reverse the process.

b: Bill is unlikely to be suffering from burnout because, although committed to his work, he has the ability to break off from it and has developed other interests. As long as the quality of his care for his patients and his management of the ward are not impaired, his hobby is a strong defence against burnout.

c: Sheila is at risk from burnout. The counselling skills she has developed are a very valuable asset to her patients and colleagues, but she is becoming too involved with the patients, sacrificing her personal life for her professional one. By concentrating on just one nursing task in this way, she may also be neglecting other duties. Hard work in preparation for exams involves only temporary commitment and, once they're over, she may be able to restore the balance a little by developing her social life and her own interests. As a student she should be able to rely on the support and care of her peers, who should see that she is under stress and give her the appropriate support.

4. You are the sister in charge of a busy intensive care unit. A new consultant is making heavy demands on your time and that of your staff, with requirements which you feel should not take priority over some other essential tasks. There is a tense atmosphere among the nurses with hostility toward the consultant and yourself, and even between themselves. What do you do?
   a) Try and set up a meeting with the consultant, yourself, and senior staff nurses.
   b) Whenever a confrontation occurs between staff, interrupt them and change the subject.
   c) Ignore the situation and try to cut yourself off.

Situation 4
a. Try and set up a meeting. Talking things over frankly and openly clears the air, and the priorities for work within the unit can be established and made clear to all. Stress the fact that you are a team, working together to help patients. Would regular meetings of this kind be of value?

Conclusion
Burnout is not a new concept, although the term may be new to our language. It is a condiiton that is perhaps being recognised more frequently, although its incidence among health care professionals may not have actually increased. Recognition of the symptoms of burnout, and those of stress, are essential in preventing the occurrence of both conditions, and in the support and treatment of their victims.

References
Cherniss, C., (1980) Staff Burnout. Sage, London.
Edelwich, J., and Brodsky, A., (1980) Burnout: Stages of Disillusionment in the Helping Professions. Human Sciences Press, London.
Niehouse, O. L., (1981) Burnout! A Real Threat to Human Resources Managers. *Personnel (USA)*, **58; 5,** 25.
Squires, A., and Livesley, B., (1984) Beware of Burnout, *Physiotherapy*, **70; 6,** p. no 235.

Proper management of intercostal drains is essential both for the patient's quick recovery and peace of mind. Many nurses are, however, confused by conflicting ideologies.

Managing intercostal drains

Mark Foss, BSc, RGN, PGCEA
Nurse Tutor, Nottingham School of Nursing

Nurses working in general medical, thoracic surgical and other wards are often involved in the care of patients who have intercostal drains and the principle of the underwater seal is covered in all basic nurse education programmes. Despite both these facts many nurses experience uncertainty in the day to day management of the intercostal drain, and conflict often arises when different ideologies are presented. This difficulty arises partly from a lack of sound reasoning and this article attempts to discuss some of the management alternatives.

---

1. Harold Smith is 62 and has chronic obstructive airways disease. He was admitted to hospital with severe chest pain and breathlessness. Chest expansion on the right side was reduced and the provisional diagnosis of pneumothorax was confirmed by chest X-ray. An intercostal drain was inserted and Mr Smith was transferred to the ward area. It was noticed that the connection between Mr Smith's chest drain and the tube to the drainage bottle was continually working loose and occasionally becoming disconnected.

Which of the following solutions should you propose?

a. Explain the problem to Mr Smith and ask him to restrict his activity so as to decrease the likelihood of disconnection.

b. Extensively tape the connection to make it secure.

c. Do nothing to secure the connection for fear of masking the join.

d. Change the connector and tubing to the drainage bottle. If this fails apply one piece of 1.5cm tape to both sides of the connection leaving the join visible from the front and back. Apply two more pieces, this time passing them around the tubing above and below the connection (Figure 1).

---

a. Maintaining maximum mobility, preventing shoulder stiffness and promoting full chest expansion are important aspects in the nursing care. Mr Smith's activity should be encouraged, especially since anxiety and discomfort will tend to reduce mobility. He could, however, be taught to check the tightness of the connection.

b. Extensively taped connections are initially secure but often work loose and disconnection may then be masked by the binding.

c. This option leaves the patient with the anxiety of a frequently broken connection and drainage of the pleural space may be delayed.

d. Changing the tubing may remedy the problem of disconnection, especially if rubber tubing is used, since this perishes with time. Taping the connection in the manner described ensures that the join is made fast but the connection remains visible.

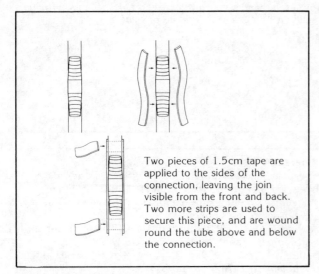

Two pieces of 1.5cm tape are applied to the sides of the connection, leaving the join visible from the front and back. Two more strips are used to secure this piece, and are wound round the tube above and below the connection.

Figure 1. Securing the connections.

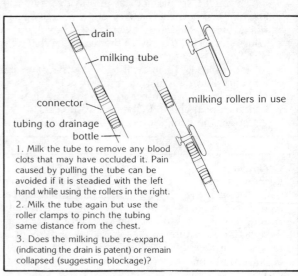

— drain

— milking tube

connector

tubing to drainage bottle

milking rollers in use

1. Milk the tube to remove any blood clots that may have occluded it. Pain caused by pulling the tube can be avoided if it is steadied with the left hand while using the rollers in the right.

2. Milk the tube again but use the roller clamps to pinch the tubing same distance from the chest.

3. Does the milking tube re-expand (indicating the drain is patent) or remain collapsed (suggesting blockage)?

Figure 2. When drainage stops.

2. After five days the bubbling from Mr Smith's chest drain remained very brisk and he was seen by a thoracic surgeon who agreed to take over his care. Mr Smith was scheduled for a pleurectomy in the local cardiothoracic centre. Upon his transfer in an ambulance which of the following options regarding the management of the chest drain would you choose?

a. Clamp the chest drain prior to moving Mr Smith.

b. Do not clamp the drain unless the closed drainage system is broken.

c. Do not clamp the drain. Should disconnection occur, simply reconnect the tubing quickly.

a. Not a good option at all. In the presence of such brisk bubbling of air from the pleural space, clamping the drain for even short periods of time may result in respiratory embarrassment as the affected lung is compressed by the accumulation of air. This may lead to mediastinal shift and its associated problems.

b. Usually the chosen option but in the presence of such brisk bubbling, clamping even for short periods of time whilst the drain is reconnected may result in respiratory difficulty and pain.

c. Definitely the best option. Rapid reconnection restores pleural drainage and avoids the possibility of the development of a positive pleural pressure as a result of clamping. For emergency use, in the event of bottle breakage, a Heimlich valve may be carried. When connected to the chest drain it will allow the one way movement of air out of the pleura.

---

3. Mr Smith undergoes a right pleurectomy and returns from theatre with apical and basal chest drains in place under 100mmHg (13KPa) suction. In the first four hours after operation 300ml of heavily blood stained drainage are noted but following this the drainage bottle measurements remain stable. With this in mind, which of the following actions do you consider to be advisable?

a. No action is required since the bleeding has obviously stopped.

b. Let the doctor know that the drainage has stopped.

c. Try to interpret the meaning of the absence of drainage. Check that the drainage tube is not kinked or compressed by the patient lying on it. Milk the drain with roller clamps and note, when the rollers are used to compress the tubing some distance from the chest, if it remains collapsed or if it re-expands (Figure 2).

a. This would be a somewhat short sighted option. Has the bleeding really stopped or is the chest drain blocked?

b. Not the best option unless you are unfamiliar with chest drains. You could intervene more fully to discover why there is no more drainage.

c. If drainage stops suddenly a kinked or blocked drain should always be considered. Milking may dislodge a blockage (a clot of blood) and observation of the tube which is pinched after milking will show whether the drain is patent or not. The patent drain will re-expand, whilst one which is blocked will remain collapsed.

---

4. After seven postoperative days you are asked to remove Mr Smith's chest drains. Which of the following alternative strategies would you choose?

a. Disconnect the drains from suction and remove them in any order.

b. Disconnect the drains from suction and remove the basal drain first. (The apical and basal drains can be differentiated from their positions on the lateral chest X-ray and from the nature of their drainage. The basal drain will primarily have drained fluid, and the apical mainly air).

c. Remove both drains under suction, the basal first.

It is advisable to remove the basal drain first since any accumulation of air in the pleura following removal of the basal drain will be evacuated through the remaining apical drain. The reverse does not apply since air in the pleura will rise to the apex of the lung. In addition there is no need to disconnect the drains from suction prior to their removal (although the suction should be reduced) and indeed the vacuum may help prevent air entering the pleura during the procedure. If both drains are connected to one bottle via a 'Y' connector, the basal drain should be clamped and removed first. The apical drain can then be removed under suction.

Bibliography

Fishman, N.H. (1983) Thoracic Drainage – A Manual Of Procedures. Year Book Medical Publishers Inc.

Foss, M.A. (1989) Thoracic Surgery. Austen Cornish Publishers Ltd, London.

MacFarlane, J. (1986) Inserting a chest drain. *Hospital Doctor*, **106**, 33, 29.

Mumford, S.P. (1986) Draining the pleural cavity. *The Professional Nurse*, **1**, 9, 240–242.

Sturridge, M.F. and Treasure, T. (1985) Belcher's Thoracic Surgical Management. Fifth Edition. Baillière Tindall.

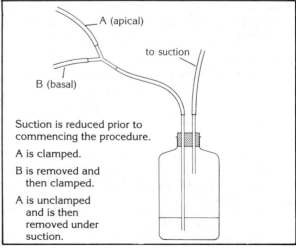

Figure 3. Removing the drains.

Incontinence is an extensive health problem which causes severe difficulties for sufferers and their families. Health care professionals must give sensitive and practical advice to minimise these difficulties and thus the misery and embarrassment incontinence can cause.

Living with incontinence

Keith Hurst, RGN, DipN, RCNT, RNT, CertEd

Senior Nurse Research, Central Nottinghamshire Health Authority and Lecturer, Nuffield Institute, Leeds University

The extent and nature of the problems of urinary and faecal incontinence in the community have been investigated in a recent research project. The main findings were as follows:

- Incontinence causes a wide range of practical, psychological and social problems for its sufferers and their families and carers.
- Lack of knowledge and understanding of their condition contributes to a sense of hopelessness and apathy in sufferers and their carers; patient education can help them to maintain an optimistic outlook.
- The care for an incontinent person at home is usually undertaken by wife, mother or daughter; men are rarely involved.
- The level of satisfaction with the various treatment methods was mixed, and the most comfortable solution was rarely found straight away.
- The use of undergarments was the most widely adopted method of overcoming incontinence.
- Where the patient or carer had evaluated the effectiveness of their method of continence care, and were involved as a result in re-assessment of treatment, then their level of satisfaction remained high.
- Fewer than half the respondents wanted to attend an incontinence clinic for specialist assessment and care.

Anyone wanting further information about this research is welcome to contact Keith Hurst at Birch House, Ransom Hospital, Mansfield, Notts NG21 0ER.

Part of the study asked people suffering from incontinence for their own view of their problems; in many cases their carers (usually wife, mother or daughter) replied on their behalf. The following situations are adapted from some of their responses. They may form a useful basis for thought or discussion.

Situation 1

'My mother is 81 and has had this problem (urinary incontinence) for three years. The cause is mostly laziness and old age. She will not try to overcome it despite being cared for by people who understand the problem (primary health care team).'

Another daughter said: 'She is not at all upset by being wet or in a mess, we have tried very hard with great kindness but it is no use. I would welcome any help finding out the real cause.'

What support is most appropriate for these two families?

These two respondents are both indicating their lack of knowledge of incontinence. Carefully planned patient education would help them to understand the problem and its solutions more fully. The situation of these two respondents contrast sharply with that of the young mother in Situation 2.

Situation 2

'Following the delivery of my third child I developed a vesico-vaginal fistula and incontinence, which, following repair, took about 10 weeks to settle down.' This young mother goes on to explain how she observed the incontinence worsening prior to, during and for a short period after menstruation.

What form of support would be of most help to her?

It is clear that this respondent had an excellent relationship with her carers, and their clear explanations of her condition had enabled her to cope with the acute episode and with her illness.

Situation 3

'My husband had a stroke three years ago and it affected his mind as well as leaving him incontinent of bowel and bladder. He is physically strong and can get around quite well if accompanied. He will not keep dry, will not co-operate at all. When asked to go to the toilet he says he doesn't want to then wets or messes himself soon after. He uses every ruse possible to remove his plastic pants and pads, hiding them in drawers with clean linen, behind the hot water cistern, in the dustbin, anywhere and everywhere. I once found a soiled pad in the breadbin! Attending hospital for treatment and care makes him worse because he dislikes going. Similarly, when I want him to do something he doesn't want to, he will wet himself. I think he does it deliberately.' Mrs Brown is 81 years old and ends her response by saying that at times she wishes she were dead.

What form of help would be of most value to this couple?

Mrs Brown clearly feels that her husband's stroke has changed him, and she now views him, and to some measure treats him, as a child. Mr Brown's apparently unco-operative behaviour may result from his refusal to accept this new identity. Discussing this with Mrs Brown may help her to view her husband as an adult, and for him to begin to accept that his lifestyle has changed in a way that will require considerable support from his wife.

Situation 4

'Tablets worked at first but no longer do so. Pads and pants leak and my clothes get ruined. I am at a loss to know what to do next so I just don't drink anything. I don't think anything more can be done.'

'I am too old for further help and I cannot be bothered with anything new. No, I would not be interested in going to a special clinic since I have seen the specialist and all help possible has been given.'

'My son has wet himself since birth. He is now 12 years old and I don't know what the cause is. We try to toilet train him, which works sometimes. I don't really know how I could be helped more.'

How can these people be helped?

Long term incontinence can make the sufferer feel a sense of resignation and even apathy towards their condition, and the active involvement of an interested carer or adviser can help to maintain the sufferer's positive outlook on their problem. If one form of treatment proves unsatisfactory, other methods can be tried.

The research project showed that this pattern of re-assessment of the patient's problem did occur, but that tried and tested methods were used first. Undergarments were the most common method of overcoming incontinence (52 per cent of patients in this survey).

Situation 5

The final part of the research attempted to determine what incontinent sufferers perceived as their main needs. The outcomes are perhaps the most disturbing of all the findings. More than half did not wish to attend an incontinence clinic for specialist assessment and care. The reason for this was that the respondent was, on the whole, satisfied with their existing pattern of care.

'No thank you. I am satisfied with the care I get from my GP and nurse.'

'I think this would be a waste of time in view of my mother's age.'

'At 92 years of age I think that my mother is best cared for at home.'

Other respondents qualified their willingness to attend:

'I wouldn't want to stay there but I would be prepared to go for one day.'

This last section poses health carers quite a problem. It is clear from the previous discussion that patients with incontinence and their carers have special needs and problems. It is also clear that the respondents are indicating to us how their needs should be met, and a hospital-based service isn't one of them. There would, however, be merit in exploring the value of a community-based continence adviser who could visit patients and carers at home to provide a personal and individualised service. Furthermore, the adviser could act as a liaison officer between patient, primary health care team, hospital and other agencies such as manufacturers of aids for the incontinent. In fact, the main recommendation arising out of this survey is the establishment of the post of a continence adviser to help relieve patients and their carers of the misery inflicted by incontinence.

Bibliography

Egan, M., Plymat, K., Thomas, T. and Mead, T. (1983) Incontinence in patients in two district general hospitals, *Nursing Times*, **79**, 5, 22-23.
A survey of the problem of incontinence in two district general hospitals, highlighting the extent and nature of the problem among inpatients.

Mandelstam, D. and Robinson, W. (1977) Support for the incontinent patient, *Nursing Mirror* supplement, xix.
Considers many aspects of incontinence and how a nurse can help the patient overcome problems.

Swaffield, L. (1981) Attitudes to incontinence, *Nursing Times* Community Outlook, 51.
Examines the attitudes of sufferers, carers and staff to the promotion of continence.

Tallis, R. and Norton, C. (1984-5) Incontinence in the elderly, *Nursing Times*. (series), **80**, 39; **80**, 44; **80**, 48; **81**, 10; **81**, 14; **81**, 18.
An extensive discussion of incontinence in the elderly, ranging from an explanation of the aetiology to the assessment, planning, implementation and evaluation of appropriate nursing care.

Each winter, hypothermia threatens the lives of many elderly people. Under some circumstances, younger, fit, and healthy people may also be at risk. It is a condition that is wholly preventable, and one that, if discovered early enough, is completely and simply reversible. Hypothermia isn't always easy to recognise, however, because its symptoms are nonspecific and can easily be mistaken for those of other disorders.

Hypothermia: one of winter's threats to the elderly

Elizabeth M. Horne, MA
Editorial Director, The Professional Nurse

'Hypothermia' literally means lower than normal body temperature. The normal, healthy body is homeothermic; that is, it maintains a reasonably constant core (internal) temperature of around 98.4°F (37°C), despite environmental changes.

Normally, if the body temperature starts to drop, nerve endings in the skin are stimulated and initiate the well-known bodily responses to the cold, including subcutaneous vasoconstriction, shivering, reduced sweat gland activity and horripilation or "goosepimpling" (raising of the hairs of the skin to trap insulating pockets of air), which together result in the production and conservation of heat within the body. The individual may also respond consciously to the sensation of cold, by moving into a warmer environment, putting on additional clothing, or increasing his or her level of exercise.

If these responses fail, or are inadequate to balance heat loss, the body's core temperature continues to drop. The subcutaneous muscles increase their demand for oxygen and produce more carbon dioxide as they increase their level of activity, and unless oxygen is supplied and carbon dioxide disposed of, carbonic and lactic acids build up and inhibit muscular activity. Shivering and vasoconstriction cease and the production and conservation of heat is reduced. This state of moderate hypothermia will deteriorate if measures are not taken to reverse it, and in severe hypothermia the body's muscles become flaccid and the individual becomes comatose. Acidosis will rapidly develop and this will affect the heart muscles causing bradycardia or tachycardia, atrial fibrillation, and ultimately cardiac arrest resulting from ventricular fibrillation. Table 1 summarises the progressively deteriorating condition of the body with increasing hypothermia.

Hypothermia may be difficult to identify, particularly if the patient is unconscious, since the symptoms are nonspecific and may look similar to those of other conditions. The most important assessment of the patient is that of his or her rectal temperature, which will give a reliable measure of the body's core temperature. Hypothermia can only be resolved by rewarming the patient and then ensuring that normal body temperature is maintained.

The following situations may help to illustrate some of the risk factors and appropriate nursing intervention

1. Who of the following is most at risk from hypothermia this February?
   (a) 64-year-old Mrs Watson, who lives in a centrally heated house and who keeps the thermostat set at around 65°F. She lives alone and has been severely depressed since her husband's death 6 months ago. She is taking regular doses of antidepressant drugs prescribed by her GP.
   (b) 75-year-old Mrs James, who is thin and spry and normally very active and who regularly cycles to the nearby village to do her shopping. She has recently broken her hip in a fall and is now unable to move very far. She usually heats her living room with a coal fire but her present condition makes carrying coal difficult.
   (c) John and Sarah Daniels, who are fit and healthy 30-year-olds whose main hobby is sailing. They particularly enjoy sailing in challenging conditions and have just set off for a holiday sailing along the Norwegian coast.

Situation 1
The elderly are particularly vulnerable to hypothermia because the normal slowing down of bodily functions that occurs with old age often results in decreased physical activity and also a diminished capacity to shiver and to regulate core temperature. In addition, elderly people living on low income may find it difficult to finance adequate heating for their homes.

(a) Mrs Watson, although she usually keeps her house at a reasonable temperature, may be at risk, because antidepressants (in common with many other drugs) produce vasodilatation and inhibit shivering. Her depressed state may also make her less aware of and interested in her own physical condition.

(b) Mrs James is clearly at risk now that she is immobile, especially since she has relatively little body fat.

(c) If John or Sarah Daniels accidentally fall into the cold waters they are sailing in, they will rapidly become hypothermic and risk quick death unless they are well protected (for example by wet-suits) and are rescued from the water quickly and gradually rewarmed. A fit adult unprotected by special clothing will live for only 5 minutes in water at freezing temperature. Other outdoor hobbies, such as camping or skiing could also result in hypothermia.

2. You make a routine visit to see Mrs Watson (see **Situation 1** above) and find her in a very confused state. She is not shivering, but her skin seems cold and her face is very pink. She says that she has not eaten much in the past few days and admits to having increased her dose of the antidepressants in the hope that she'll feel better. She had turned the central heating down earlier in the week in an economy drive. Her rectal temperature is 90°F (32°C). Would you:

(a) Set the central heating to a higher level (say 68°F (20°C) and wrap her in warm blankets?

(b) Help her to take a warm bath?

(c) Give her several hot water bottles?

(d) Make her some warm and nutritious soup?

(e) Help her to plan a reasonable strategy for keeping warm in the future?

Situation 2

Mrs Watson clearly needs to be rewarmed to her normal body temperature. Her core temperature is so low that option **(a)**, *passive warming*, relying upon her body's ability to generate the heat required to restore normal body temperature, may not be sufficient, and **(b)** *active warming*, by gradually applying warmth externally, may be required. Hot water bottles **(c)** should not be used; care must be taken not to burn Mrs Watson, nor to cause vasodilatation of the capillaries in her skin which would divert warm blood to the peripheries and away from central body organs, causing a drop in core temperature. She should be rewarmed gradually; any attempt to apply sudden heat will result in a drop in core temperature. **(d)** A warming drink will assist in restoring her normal core temperature, but, more importantly, her nutritional status needs improving with a gradual return to well-balanced and regular eating habits. **(e)** Once she is rewarmed, reasonably fed, and feeling better, advice and support with a strategy for keeping warm in the future will be essential; it may be difficult for her to co-operate with and respond positively to this because of her depressed state, and if this proves to be a continuing problem, her GP may consider referring her for psychiatric treatment.

3. Your next visit is to Mrs James, whom you find unconscious in her extremely cold living room. There is no fire lit and she is wearing a thin woollen dress. Her respiration rate is extremely low and you cannot detect a pulse at all. Her rectal temperature is 86°F (30°C). Would you:

(a) Wrap her in warm blankets with hot water bottles; light a fire and warm the living room?

(b) Arrange for her to be admitted to the local hospital, where she is given a warmed oxygen inhalation?

(c) In the medium term, arrange for local Social Services workers to visit Mrs James and assess her requirement for a more reliable source of heating and, if necessary, meals?

(d) Once Mrs James is back home, discuss and plan with her a strategy for staying warm?

Situation 3

Mrs James' core temperature has dropped so low that **(b)** *internal warming* will be essential to restore her normal core temperature. External warming **(a)** would not be sufficient. **(c)** and **(d)** In the medium term she clearly needs help with a strategy for keeping warm.

Rectal temperature	Symptoms of hypothermia	Precipitating factors
98° - 95°F (37° - 35°C)	Shivering Horripilation Cold, pale skin Poor muscle coordination Hyperpnoea Tachycardia	*Social:* Exposure to cold; Isolation; Poverty; Poor diet; Inadequate heating. Impairment of the heat-regulating mechanism
95° - 90°F (35° - 32°C)	Cold skin Waxy appearance Pink and puffy face Confusion No shivering Bradypnoea	*Endocrine:* Myxaoedema; Diabetes; Hypopituitarism *Mental:* Dementia; Confusion
90° - 86°F (32° - 30°C)	Rigid muscles Dilated pupils Poor reflexes Coma Low blood pressure Bradycardia	*Immobility:* Falls; Arthritis; Parkinsonism; Strokes *Drugs:* Phenothiazines; Alcohol;
86° - 82°F (30° - 28°C)	Coma Flaccid muscles Bradycardia or tachycardia Fixed, dilated pupils Atrial fibrillation Possible cardiac arrest	Antidepressants; Barbiturates; Hypnotics *Illness:* Infections; Stroke;
82° - 68°F (28° - 20°C)	Cyanosis Barely detectable vital signs Cardiac arrest	Myocardial infarction; Septicaemia

Table 1: The symptoms of deepening hypothermia

Table 2: Preventing hypothermia: advice to elderly patients

- Put on extra layers of clothes, particularly when going out of doors in cold weather. Several thinner layers provide more insulation than one thick garment. Don't forget to wear a hat, especially if your hair is thin

- Eat nutritious meals and have hot drinks regularly

- Try to keep the rooms you live and sleep in warm; if you can only afford to heat one room, have your bed moved into the living room that you do heat. Try not to make economies with your fuel bills and seek help from social services or your family and friends if paying your fuel bill is difficult

- Wear socks and a cap in bed and use an electric blanket or hot water bottle to warm your bed before bedtime

- Don't over-exert yourself, but do try to move around during the day

- Take warm baths only and dry yourself thoroughly afterwards, to prevent heat loss as the excess water evaporates

Do you agree that if a patient wishes, they have the right to know about, and understand, their illness and its treatment? How good are you at giving information? Do you find it difficult to answer painful questions? Do you ever ignore, or pay scant attention to, a question you consider to be trivial — especially when you are busy? Do you always make yourself understood?

Giving verbal information

Janet Gooch, SRN, Dip.N(Lond), RCNT
Ward Sister, Brighton General Hospital

What information is needed? Nurses are continually giving out information to a wide variety of people but this does not necessarily mean that they always give the information people would like to have. Research findings support the supposition that very often they do not. Many of the complaints received about nursing care appear to centre around a lack of information and communication.

Clearly we have to learn what information it is that people really want — and find ways to ensure that they receive it. Obviously the best people to tell us what information is required are those seeking it — patients, their relatives, and our colleagues. Perhaps we should ask *them?*.

Having asked, we should learn to listen actively to the replies. Only then are we likely to recognise and understand correctly what has been said and to respond in the necessary way.

How is information to be given? In the same way that there is little point in a nurse asking a question unless they are prepared to listen to the answer, it is pointless to give replies that the questioner cannot understand. To ensure effective understanding it is essential to use a common language. Nursing and medical staff are notorious for the use of their own specialised language which is largely incomprehensible to the outsider. Jargonese should be avoided where it could be a barrier to understanding.

The emphasis and tone of voice in which something is said can express a meaning as much as the words used.

For instance "I will come and tell you later" can be changed from a promise to a brush off merely by the tone of voice, emphasis placed on different words, set of the lips, facial expression, and body stance.

If patients and relatives are not given the information they want by the appropriate person then they must seek it elsewhere. Other patients, domestic staff, porters, and very junior nurses can all seem approachable and non-threatening. If they also show that they have more time to talk than trained staff then they are the ones who will probably be asked to answer questions. This may well be appropriate, but in many instances their replies may be misleading, or at worst totally inaccurate. The obvious way to avoid this is for trained staff to be the first people to show themselves as available and ready to answer questions, to inform, and to listen.

Furthermore, silence can be construed as an answer to either spoken or unspoken questions. The patient who asks to be informed of the result of his blood test may presume the result is too bad for him to be told if the nurse forgets to return to him with the information he requested.

Sharing information with colleagues: Nurses have not only to communicate with patients and relatives, but also to pass information to each other. Verbal reports on patients' condition and treatment, teaching learners, counselling, and discussions are examples of when information is given. If the information given is faulty what may the outcome be?

The following situations could form the basis for discussion between yourself and colleagues.

Situation 1
A patient calls you over to his bed to tell you that his wife is worried about something. Would you reply:
a) "Well, tell her to come and see me"?
b) "What is she worried about?"
c) "Don't you worry about that now"?
d) "Is there anything I can do to help?"

b) and **d)** would both allow the patient to express his worries and tell you what information he really wants. He may have found it easier to blame his anxiety on his wife than to admit to his own fears. The only way to know is to make it easy for him to talk to you.

Situation 2
You overhear a patient telling his wife that no-one has told him what is wrong. You yourself have explained to the patient about his condition and that he is waiting for special X-rays. Should you:

a) Ignore it?

c) Would seem ideal but either the patient has decided not to tell his wife what he knows or he did not understand the information. In the latter case to repeat what you have already said would be pointless.

d) In this way you can find out exactly what *he* wants to know and give him information appropriate to his need. You may find out that previously you had told him only what *you*

---

b) Go to the bedside and tell the wife that you have in fact explained everything to him that morning?

c) Go and sit with them both and give them the information again?

d) Sit with the patient again after his wife has left and discover what he has understood so far and what else he wants to know, ask him if he would like you to give his wife the information?

e) Make a point of speaking to the wife on her next visit and offer to answer any questions?

wanted him to know. Offering to give the information to his wife will establish whether he wishes her to know about his condition.

e) Would be very valuable as long as the patient's confidentiality is not being breached in your replies.

Situation 3

Preoperatively Mr Harrison insists that whatever is found at operation he himself should not be told. He asks that whatever information needs to be imparted should be given to his wife. When asked what he thinks is wrong with him he says that he knows he has an ulcer in his stomach. He appears extremely tense, avoids eye contact, and speaks to staff only in reply to questions. After surgery to remove successfully a gastric cancer his postoperative recovery is marred by his poor emotional state. He complains about various symptoms such as constipation, nausea, and weakness but refuses to listen to any explanation of these problems. When the time comes for his discharge he delays this by saying that he does not feel ready.

In discussion with Mrs Harrison she agrees that her husband was worrying that he was dying of cancer. She herself would like her husband to be told that the surgery had removed the tumour but had acceded to their daughter's ban on this. What would most help the patient.

a) Telling him exactly what was found at operation and explaining the probable success of the procedure?

b) Knowing how much Mr Harrison relied on his wife, trying to persuade their daughter to allow Mrs Harrison to tell her husband what she felt he wanted to know?

c) Asking the doctor to give the information about the diagnosis?

d) Discussing with Mr Harrison the reasons why he did not want to know about his condition?

Mr Harrison clearly needs some information to help him deal with his feelings. If he is unwilling to ask direct questions about his condition, or to express his anxiety, even if given plenty of opportunity and encouragement to do so, then option **(b)** involving his family, and perhaps **(c)** involving the doctor (if it is felt that Mr Harrison may prefer to discuss his condition with medical staff), may prove helpful. **(d)** Encouraging him to talk about his reasons for not wanting to know may enable him to express his fear of cancer and of death, and for these anxieties then to be dispelled. Unless this problem is exposed, Mr Harrison may not believe any encouraging information given to him because he may feel that everyone is being kind *because* his fears are justified.

Situation 4

Nurse Woods is given a verbal report about her patient Mr Steel in which she is told that after an attack of severe chest pain and hypotension he has been diagnosed as having a pulmonary embolism. A short time later the patient is missing from his bed and is found in the bath having been taken there by Nurse Woods, who has herself gone to coffee. In this situation:

a) Why might Nurse Woods have responded to the report in this way?

b) How could it be ensured that such an incident is not likely to be repeated?

a) The senior nurses present at the report all understood the gravity of Mr Steel's condition but failed to ensure that the learners shared that knowledge. Nurse Woods was asked at the end of the report whether she had any questions but she thought she knew what pulmonary embolism meant so did not realise her need to check that understanding. The report was hurried because the night nurse was late going off duty and she did not mention that Mr Steel was confined to bed — she had presumed that this fact was obvious.

b) It is essential that when any piece of information is imparted it is known to have been correctly interpreted and understood. Had Nurse Woods been asked to state what she understood about pulmonary embolisms and what implications that diagnosis had for the patient, her lack of knowledge would have become known. She could then have been informed and the patient not put at risk.

Conclusion

Giving instructions and advice is not the same thing as giving information that a person wants and needs to receive. Information must be given at the time the patient is ready to receive it. The only way to avoid errors of understanding is to give information freely when it is needed, and to ensure that both words and attitudes have made the meaning clear.

Bibliography

Bridge, W., and Macleod Clark, J. (1981) Communication in Nursing Care. HM&M, London.
A collection of many of the factors and issues involved when nurses communicate with patients.

Hewitt, F.S. (1981) Communication skills. *Nursing Times* (Occasional Papers), July 16, August 26.
Discusses the dynamics of giving information.

Reynolds, M. (1978) No news is bad news: Patient's views about communication. *British Medical Journal*, **i**, 1673.

What do you know about AIDS and HIV? What do you feel about the subject? This Practice Check and the one which follows it are to help you explore your own feelings about this difficult subject, and the ethical issues which surround it.

Test your approach towards AIDS/HIV

James Stanford, BA, RGN, DN
Community Nurse, Brighton Health Authority

Studies have shown that despite the high profile AIDS has had in the mass media and in the nursing press, there is still a high level of misunderstanding, misinformation and prejudice surrounding it. The subject of AIDS and HIV involves many issues which merit attention. There are many areas which are still not well understood both by members of the public and by many nurses. Below are five situations which highlight a number of issues that relate to this topic. The points made against each situation are in no way exhaustive. Many other issues may be usefully explored when analysing each situation. The points made are merely an aid to further discussion. The characters in these examples are fictitious, their names being taken from the works of Henry James.

---

1. Duty to the patient

Morris Townsend is a 19-year-old man who has been admitted to Daffodil ward where you are the nurse in charge. He is estranged from his parents, whom he has not seen for two years. He requests that his lover, Owen, should be recorded as his next of kin. Morris has pneumocystis pneumonia and is terminally ill. His mother rings for information. What would you do?

- The first line of action must be to inform Morris that his mother has telephoned and to ask him what information he wishes her to be given.
- Our first duty as nurses is to the patient. If Morris asks that his mother is not told the full details of his illness, his wishes must be respected. As he is over 18 years old, he is an adult and his parents have no legal control over him or legal access to personal information that he may wish to withold.

---

2. The patient's consent

Maisie Farange is a 23-year-old woman who has been run over by a car. She has been admitted to A&E with multiple injuries and may require surgery. She is fully conscious and alert and asks for her parents to be informed of her accident. The casualty officer notices puncture marks on her left arm and asks you to take a blood specimen for HIV antibodies without consent. What would your reaction be? If consent is sought, but refused, what then would your reaction be?

- Before being tested for HIV antibodies, informed consent must be given by the person concerned. Testing without consent would be unethical.
- The BMA has suggested that HIV antibody testing could be carried out at the discretion of the doctor and without necessarily seeking the patient's consent. However, the DHSS Chief Medical Officer has not supported this stance. The UKCC has made it clear that nurses "expose themselves to the possibility of civil action for damages or criminal charges for assault being brought against them if they personally take blood samples for HIV testing without the patient's consent, and of aiding and abetting such an assault if they knowingly collude with a doctor in obtaining such specimens. In addition, they would risk allegations of misconduct" (UKCC, 1988).
- Acting as the patient's advocate, nurses need to challenge doctors who attempt to obtain blood for testing without consent. If necessary, they should refuse to assist the doctor in such a procedure, having informed their line manager.
- Maisie does in fact suffer from leukaemia and has just had a series of blood tests taken; she has not mentioned this fact and did not realise the significance that the medical staff placed on her phlebotomy wounds.

3. Needle stick injuries

Mr Longdon, aged 43, was admitted to Daffodil ward yesterday for investigations into unexplained weight loss and abdominal pain. Staff Nurse Miller has just given him an injection of i.m. pethidine, when she slips on the floor on her way to the sluice to dispose of the syringe. The unsheathed needle pierces her thumb as she falls. What action might you take as the nurse in charge?

- Ensure that Nurse Miller immediately washes her wound under running water and encourages bleeding.
- Nurse Miller may need to be seen by the occupational nurse or the casualty doctor, according to health authority policy.
- Fill out the appropriate accident form and inform the clinical nurse manager, according to policy.
- Mr Longdon's serological status regarding both hepatitis B and HIV is unknown. If he were antibody-positive to either virus, Nurse Miller's chances of contracting HIV would be negligible and of hepatitis B, low. Some health authorities recommend staff to have a hepatitis B and a tetanus vaccine, and possibly antibiotic therapy after needle stick injuries.
- The main problem here was the position of the sharps container which should have been by the bed side rather than at the far end of the ward. While it may not be practical to provide every patient with their own sharps container, patients being given frequent injections should be so provided. For other patients, the nurse should take the container to the syringe, not vice versa.
- Needles should not be resheathed or broken. Many sharps accidents occur when needles are resheathed. Even if Nurse Miller had resheathed her needle, a sharps injury was likely to occur in this instance.

4. Nursing staff fears

Kate Croy, a 47-year-old married staff nurse on Daffodil ward comes to talk to you, the nurse in charge, in the ward office. She explains she is unwilling to look after Morris Townsend as her husband is concerned that "she might catch the virus". What would your response be?

- A nurse's risk of contracting HIV infection during the course of duty is very low, but nurses do need to follow the appropriate guidelines. Even when accidents do occur, the risk of infection is very low.
- There is no reason why healthy personnel should be excused from caring for patients with AIDS/HIV related disease. The RCN has stressed that "there is no opt-out clause" (RCN, 1986) and a refusal could result in disciplinary procedures. However, there are a few exceptions. For their own wellbeing, staff with eczema should not have direct care of patients with HIV infection, neither should pregnant staff, because of the risk of transmission of cytomegalovirus (CMV) and its possible harm to the foetus. It is also common sense that staff with a current infection such as a heavy cold should not look after these or any patients.
- Kate Croy's own fears need to be explored, as well as her family's concern. Her husband's attitude may well affect her attitude towards Morris Townsend. Sexual worries may be developing between Kate and her husband. There may be conflict with colleagues. The mental stress that she may be experiencing could be an indication for the need of a staff support group.

5. Prejudice

Robert Acton is a 37-year-old district enrolled nurse in Anytown where you are a community clinical nurse manager. He is a conscientious nurse who is well liked by colleagues and patients alike. His team leader informs you that she knows Robert is gay and that he has told her that he has just found out that he is HIV-antibody-positive. She tells you that she thinks Robert has got what he deserved and that "now he's got AIDS he must be a health risk to patients". What action might you take?

- Robert is likely to be in need of help and support. It would be wise to interview him to offer counselling and reassure him about your support.
- Robert's team leader will also need support and education. Her fears of contamination and knowledge of HIV/AIDS need to be explored, as do her attitudes about homosexuality.
- A risk to his patients? As with many other illnesses, someone who is infected should be able to work as normal while medically fit to do so. Their statutory rights against unfair dismissal are not affected (DoE, 1987). "There is no evidence available to suggest that transmission of the virus from health care provider to patient has ever taken place. The possibility of this happening is probably even less likely than transmission from patient to health care provider" (RCN, 1986).
- A positive blood test for HIV antibodies indicates previous infection with the virus. It does not indicate that the person has AIDS or will necessarily develop AIDS.

References

D.o.E. and Health and Safety Executive (1987) Aids and employment.
RCN (1986) Nursing Guidelines, second report. RCN, London.

UKCC (1988) Register, January, p3. UKCC, London.

This Practice Check follows on from the previous Check and will enable you to explore further some of the thorny issues which arise in the care of patients with AIDS and HIV infection.

AIDS/HIV: how do you react?

James Stanford, BA, RGN, DN
Community Nurse, Brighton Health Authority

The ramifications of HIV infection are wide reaching. They have encompassed social, sexual, moral and medical issues, and reactions are often unnecessarily severe. Much anxiety has been fuelled by people being unsure how the virus is transmitted. As nurses, we need to be sure of the modes of transmission and how to protect ourselves and others. Our aims should be to provide the optimum care and emotional support needed by people who are, or are suspected to be, infected with the virus.

---

1. Depression

Adam Verver, aged 25, has been diagnosed as being HIV antibody positive. Recently he attended the surgery complaining of rapid weight loss and a chest infection. He is under the medical care of his GP, Dr Sloper, who is going to refer him on to a hospital consultant as soon as he can. Mr Verver appears depressed and, while you (the practice nurse) are taking a blood specimen, tells you that he is not keen to be admitted for treatment. He feels this would be a waste of time as he is sure that he will "soon be dead anyway". How do you react?

- Mr Verver's depressed state of mind may be the result of his interpretation of his current condition and prognosis. Allowing him time to voice his worries and fears will help identify what most concerns him. While it would be wrong to give him false assurances, it should be possible to give him constructive support and assistance. He may benefit from referral to a counsellor.

- Infection with HIV itself does not necessarily make someone ill, though there is a potential for illness in the future which is difficult to predict. One possible outcome of HIV infection is the development of AIDS, which may be an episodic illness; when the infections and tumours are not present, the person may be relatively well. Particularly in the early stages of the syndrome, many of the infections and some of the tumours are easily treatable, especially if diagnosed and treated rapidly. Effective treatment can greatly improve the quality and duration of life enjoyed.

- The handling of all blood, regardless of its antibody status, must be undertaken with care. Gloves should be worn when taking any blood specimen. The needle should be disposed of immediately after being removed from the syringe and placed in a sharps container without being resheathed. Next, fill the specimen jar and place the syringe in the sharps container. If the patient is known to be HIV antibody positive, a specific biohazard label may be in use in your health authority.

---

2. Withdrawal

Basil Ransom, a 63-year-old man, is being nursed in the community and is aware that he has AIDS. He has become increasingly withdrawn socially and now rarely sees any friends. Although he is capable of undertaking all activities of daily living for himself, he shows no interest in the running of his flat, which has become uncharacteristically untidy, and his appearance is now unkempt. Basil confides to you (his district nurse) that he feels useless and wishes "it was all over". How might you respond to this admission?

- Mr Ransom needs help to express his fears and anxieties. Time must be given to counsel him.
- When people become patients, they often adopt the 'sick role'. This can involve a loss of independence, social status and responsibility, and we need to help them to regain control of their lives. They need "a sympathetic understanding of themselves as a person, and someone to help them set up and plan objectives in their remaining life, recognising the limitations imposed by the disease and deciding together the help needed to achieve the maximum quality of life" (Pugsley and Pardoe, 1986).
- Because AIDS can be a fatal illness, it is easy to forget that as well as dying from the disease, people are also *living* with it. If we, as nurses, have only this perception of the illness, it could help to create an expectation of dependency and imminent death in both carer and patient.

3. Pregnancy

Olive Chancellor is a 16-year-old girl who has come to the antenatal clinic where you are a midwife. She is three months pregnant. Olive tells you that she is worried she may have contracted HIV. What issues might you need to discuss with her?

- Discover why she is concerned about HIV. The range of concerns could be quite wide, ranging from rape to overseas travel. Below we explore just a few issues.
- Enquire if there is a history of drug taking and whether she ever shares needles. The sharing of syringes and needles is a major source of HIV infection between intravenous drug users.
- It would be beneficial to discuss any drug habits her sexual partner/s may have and, any concern she may have as to who her boyfriend/s have slept with in the past.
- If she is HIV antibody positive the implications for her own health and that of her foetus need to be given serious consideration. A significant proportion of children born to mothers who are antibody positive during pregnancy will themselves be antibody positive and some will go on to develop AIDS. Pregnancy can also increase the risk to an antibody positive woman of developing AIDS.

4. Public education

You are a district nurse team leader in Anytown. The secretary of the Anytown parents' support group asks you to give a talk on AIDS/HIV to their youth club. How might you structure such an event?

- Familiarise yourself with the group characteristics, such as the size of the group and their age range, and with the overall programme. Are they having other visits from professionals on related topics, such as drug abuse, sex education or building relationships? Where would your teaching come into the programme?
- Know your resources. These might include the health authority health promotion department, local AIDS helplines, and national organisations such as the Terrence Higgins Trust and AVERT.
- Simply lecturing to a group can be of limited use in health promotion – the use of group participation and small group discussion is often more successful. Interest is more likely to be stimulated if the audience is actively involved in the session.
- A useful format can be to discover what the audience know already about AIDS/HIV and what they hope to learn from the session. One way to achieve this is to ask them to each write down three things they have heard about AIDS/HIV and to mark whether these are true, false or unsure. Then get them to share this information in small groups, and finally with the group as a whole. This will help you identify areas of concern and misconception. Meanwhile, list the main points that have been raised by the audience and then use them as the structure for the discussion with the whole group (AVERT, 1987).
- Have your own check list prepared of points you want to see covered during the session. You may find many are raised by the group.

5. Nursing procedures

You are the nurse in charge on a medical ward in a country hospital that has never before admitted a patient with AIDS/HIV infection, and your health authority has yet to publish guidelines on the nursing of such patients. You inform your clinical nurse manager that a Mr Strether arrived yesterday on the ward with an actute asthma attack, and has told you that he is HIV antibody positive. The clinical nurse manager insists that he be transferred to an isolation room and be barrier nursed with 'the full works' including masks, gowns, disposable crockery and so on. What is your reaction to this demand?

- It would be advisable for you to inform your clinical nurse manager of the facts concerning HIV transmission and the nursing of such patients. She or he may benefit from reading the RCN's Nursing Guidelines. (RCN, 1986).
- Most patients who are, or are suspected to be, HIV antibody positive, may be nursed safely in an open ward. Single room isolation is only indicated if the patient is bleeding, has an infection risk such as a pulmonary infection, or is unable to practise good hygiene, eg due to faecal incontinence, profuse diarrhoea or mental disturbance or confused behaviour that is secondary to central nervous system involvement.
- Ordinary crockery and cutlery can be used and will not need special treatment; hot soapy water is sufficient when washing up. Reusable bedpans, the ward bath, toilets and so on can be used for a patient who is HIV antibody positive – decontamination of infected articles is not difficult. A number of chemicals and detergents including hypochlorite solution (Melzone) or domestic bleach will inactivate HIV. Indeed the virus is not very infectious and is easily destroyed outside the body.

Continued over the page

6. Resuscitation

You have just finished work and are walking home when you notice a crowd has anxiously gathered around a fallen figure. You rush up to see a man collapsed and apparently unconscious. When taking his pulse, which is weak and thready you notice that his ears are pierced. Within a minute his breathing has stopped and his pulse is no longer palpable. What do you do?

- The best course of action would be to ask a member of the public to summon an ambulance. Next, ensure that his airway is clear and that he is not bleeding from his mouth. Then commence mouth to mouth resuscitation and cardiac compression until either he starts to breathe and a pulse returns or the ambulance crew arrive and take over from you. No cases of HIV transmission via saliva have been reported. There is no evidence to suggest that mouth to mouth resuscitation would place one at any risk. If there was blood present, however, there would be a risk of infection from the blood.

- Is there any significance in men wearing earrings? Would an earring lead you to draw a conclusion about a man's sexuality? If you decided he might be gay, would you then be concerned that he might also be HIV positive? Would you then be wary of contact with his body fluids? The safest course of action is to treat *everyone's* body fluids with respect – particularly blood. All blood is potentially infectious, not only with HIV, but with hepatitis B and numerous other viruses.

References

RCN (1986) Nursing Guidelines on the Management of Patients in Hospital and the Community suffering from AIDS. Second report of the RCN AIDS Working Party.

Pugsley, R. and Pardoe, J. (1986) Community care of the terminally ill patient In: Wilkes, E. (ed) Terminal Care. Update Postgraduate Centre Series, Update-Siebert, Guildford.

AVERT (1987) Learning About AIDS. AVERT, Horsham.

RCN (1986) Nursing Guidelines, second report. RCN, London.

Tatchell, P. (1986) AIDS: A Guide to Survival. Heretic Books, GMP, London.
A good general reader.

Bibliography

HEA (1987) AIDS: What Everybody Needs to Know. Health Education Authority, London.
Pamphlet with details on 'safer sex'.

Miller, D., Weber, J. and Green, J. (1986) The Management of AIDS Patients. Macmillan, London.
Medical information and practical nursing guidance.

Altman, D. (1986) AIDS and the New Puritanism. Pluto Press, London.
The political and social implications of HIV/AIDS.

Pratt, R. (1986) AIDS: A Strategy for Nursing Care. Edward Arnold, London.
Written specifically for nurses.

Acknowledgement

Thanks to Pat Evans of Brighton Health Authority Health Promotion Department for her assistance.

Useful Addresses

Terrence Higgins Trust, 52–54 Grays Inn Rd., London WC1X 8LT. Telephone: 01-833 2971.

AIDS Virus Education and Research Trust (AVERT), P.O. Box 91, Horsham, West Sussex, RH13 7YR. Telephone: 0403 864010.

Most nurses support the idea of working in partnership with patients but in practice it involves re-examining some fundamental beliefs about the nature of nursing.

Partnership with patients?

Kevin Teasdale, MA, Cert Ed., RMN

Director of In-Service Training, Pilgrim Hospital, Boston, Lincs.

How do you react when a nurse refers to patients as 'clients' or 'consumers'? Is it just jargon, or is she trying to tell you something about a belief in patients as partners in nursing care?

Partnership in nursing means an equal and adult relationship between nurse and patient. It allows for the training and expertise of the nurse, but acknowledges that the patient is also an expert on himself and his needs. It embodies the idea of a contract between the nurse and the patient. This implies that the nurse has a right and a duty to put her knowledge and skills at the disposal of the patient, but that the patient has a right and a duty to retain overall responsibility for himself and his health. An equal partnership with all patients is not possible — some do not wish to be involved in their care, some are not capable of taking in the information needed to make informed choices. But if one accepts the role of the nurse as that of helping another person to live or die as independently as possible, then the principle of partnership must be an ideal to aim at in all aspects of nursing care.

Use the following as a framework for discussion of your own nursing practice.

---

1. The principle of partnership

Partnership is a complex idea. It is easy to believe that the nurses you work with automatically accept your own view of this concept. Consider the following statements of opinion. Decide which one comes closest to your idea of partnership, and decide how you would argue for or against each of the interpretations given.

a. "Patients cannot be partners because they do not have the knowledge and skills which I acquired through training. I am the one who is accountable for what happens to them."

b. "Patients should be kept informed of what nurses are doing for them, but the final decision on nursing care rests with the nurses. If everyone was allowed to say what they wanted there would be chaos."

c. "Each patient has a right to become involved as a partner in nursing care to the extent that the patient wishes or is able to be involved."

d. "All patients must be given full information and their wishes must be met at all times."

The four statements show a range of opinion, from beliefs which allow little room for involvement of patients to those which leave little authority to the nurses.

a. Here the nurse emphasises the training which she received in making her an expert in nursing care. No allowance is made for the individuality of patients. Would a nurse who became a patient be allowed any say in her own care? The statement about accountability implies that the nurse can see no limits to her accountability, and that patients give up all responsibility for themselves.

b. This implies that patients might for example be told about the nursing care planned for them, but have no rights to influence that care. The tendency will be to permit involvement until it becomes a problem for the nurses, when attitudes will change and choices will be withdrawn. Sometimes partnership is mistaken for the idea that the patient has a right to whatever he wants, whenever he wants it. Yet the idea of equality allows the nurse to present advice, and to veto some choices, particularly when they interfere with the rights of other patients to have access to nursing resources.

c. This allows the right of involvement to the patient. It places limits on it which are concerned with the patient's capacity for responsible decision-making and communication of those decisions. It also allows for the case of the patient who says he wants no involvement. The difficult decisions are particularly those involved in deciding who is and who is not 'responsible'.

d. This implies that the 'customer is always right'. It does not acknowledge the right of the nurse to give professional advice, nor her duty to act in accord with the Code of Professional Conduct. Also it does not recognise that the rights of one patient may affect those of another.

Continued over the page

2. Facing the dilemmas

Partnership for patients is about their right to make *choices*. In order to make informed and rational choices they must also have access to *information*, and be allowed the freedom to act on their decisions. It is easy to give someone a choice when the information is clear-cut and the patient can be relied on to choose what you want him to choose. But it is not always like that. The following are examples of some of the dilemmas which will arise when nurses try to make the principle of partnership into a reality. They may lead you to think of similar situations which you have faced. Discuss how a nurse who is using a partnership approach should act in each situation.

a. A patient has returned from exploratory abdominal surgery, which has revealed inoperable cancer. The patient asks the ward sister what was the result of the operation.

b. An elderly patient who is terminally ill is confined to bed and is at risk of developing pressure sores. When the nurses come to turn him, he tells them that he doesn't want to be moved any more because it is so painful.

c. A Jehovah's Witness in a four-bed ward upsets another patient having a blood transfusion by telling him that he should not permit this.

d. In a ward where care plans and nursing notes are kept at the bedside, a patient complains that he has not been given the bath he was promised in his care plan. The primary nurse explains that there was a medical emergency on the ward, and offers to help him have a bath after lunch. The patient continues to complain.

a. Does the sister have the authority to answer? Most British nurses would probably say that the consultant has the right to control information about diagnosis and prognosis. Is this one of the situations where an equal partnership is, at least temporarily, impossible? Each situation would have to be assessed on its merits, and most nurses and doctors would agree that skill and thought is also needed in selecting the right time and place to give information or explain choices. However if partnership is seen as fundamental to nursing care, it follows that there should always be a bias towards truth-giving, unless sound arguments to the contrary can be found.

b. Partnership requires that full information on the risk of pressure sores be given if the person is able to understand it. Then a negotiation must take place which respects the right of the fully informed patient to choose. The nurse must try to agree a decision with the patient which is rational and compassionate. This may mean discussion over use of a ripple bed or a water bed, with the patient understanding that these may not be as effective in prevention of pressure sores as regular turning. It might involve the patient in monitoring pain levels.

c. The adult Jehovah's Witness has a right to his own opinions and to be nursed according to his wishes. However he has no right to interfere in the professional relationship between health care staff and other patients, and this must be made clear to him.

d. Open access to information tends to reduce complaints by promoting good communication. In this case, the nurse must record correctly what the patient said and her reply, then show it to the patient. The nurse's duty is thus to listen to what the patient is saying, do what she can to meet his needs, and explain any reasons why she cannot do this completely as the patient wishes. But the principle of partnership recognises the right of the nurse to organise nursing resources to benefit all the patients in her care. Persistent complaints are usually less about the problem itself, than about the way the complaint was handled. Open access to nursing records proves to the patient that his complaint has been heard.

3. Principles into practice

Consider your own nursing practice in the following areas. What are you doing at present which supports the patient's right to involvement as a partner, and what more could be done?

a. *Verbal information* — exactly what is the patient told by nurses on first contact, during the period of nursing care, and before discharge? What is the patient not told? How are handovers managed?

b. *Written information* — can the patient see his care plan? Is anything written on the forms which is not available to the patient? Do relatives and friends have access to written information?

c. How many *choices* may the patient make each day? In which activities does the patient have choices, and in which does he not?

Continued opposite

a. *Verbal information* — many care plans will state: "explain the admission procedure and ward layout", but lack any instruction to check whether what was said was understood. In some hospital wards nurses try to ensure a coherent approach to information-giving by having written booklets available for patients. Handover systems vary, but a bedside handover may help to involve and inform the patient as well as the nurses. Specific items of confidential information may be given at the nurses' station. It takes skill and practice to get each patient talking and at ease.

b. *Written information* — what will happen if care plans are kept at the bedside? In principle, if involvement is sought, then the patient must see what is written. Most patients will not look at care plans even at the bedside unless specifically given permission to do so. Fears that relatives or friends may see are often exaggerated. A bedside wallet will keep away prying eyes. Whatever is written should be factual rather than opinion. The danger with separate forms at the nurses' station is that they become another nursing Kardex and devalue care plans. But, in gynaecological areas for example, patients may prefer that some information be stored away from the bedside.

c. *Choices* — the key to partnership. Essentially it involves negotiation. Getting up in the morning for example. If all the patients want to get up at 9am the nurses will be unable to cope. But partnership approaches encourage nurses to involve patients through agreeing compromises between their wishes and the limits on the resources available. Some nursing models lend themselves to this approach by emphasising the educative, facilitative role of the nurse.

d. If the care plans all disappeared tomorrow, would it make any difference to the way in which you and the other nurses give nursing care? In other words, how much of your care is routine, and how much of it develops from a partnership between nursing knowledge and patients' wishes?

d. *Planned partnership* — ideas such as:
- Do any of the care plans show contracts? For example that the nurse will teach the patient a breathing and relaxation technique, then the patient will use this regularly after the operation, and keep a record of pain levels to help in planning further pain management.
- How many rules do patients have to accept without question in your area? When were the reasons for these rules last examined?
- Have you considered open visiting, or self-medication for patients? What would be the benefits, as well as the disadvantages?

4. Making it happen

To make partnership a reality you need to understand the *content* — what the patients want from the service — and the *process* — ways in which change may be facilitated. Consider the following questions as challenges to help you determine a plan for constructive development of partnership approaches in your own area.

a. How can you find out whether or not patients in your own clinical area are satisfied with their present level of involvement in nursing care?
b. How will you decide which aspects of patient care are top priority for moving towards a partnership approach?
c. What will be the reactions of your colleagues, nurse managers, and non-nurse colleagues to partnership approaches? What can you do to influence those reactions?
d. How could you evaluate whether or not what you are doing is having the desired effect?

a. The obvious answer is to *ask* the patients. But getting a useful answer depends on what and how you ask. If you ask hospital patients if they are satisfied with nursing care, 95 per cent will say they are very satisfied and the nurses are very busy and dedicated. If you want to get a clearer picture you must ask specific questions. "Thinking about how you felt before your operation, were there any questions you really wanted to ask but didn't feel able to?" Consumer research predicts that lack of information will be a major cause of dissatisfaction for many hospital patients.

b. You may feel very strongly that what you really want to do is to get the ward sister, consultant or GP to be more open with patients about diagnosis and prognosis. This will rarely be successful in the short term, since the change needed concerns not only communication skills, but also fundamental beliefs about health care and the role of the professional. Better to begin with something specific, and under your own control. Can any changes be made in the patients' day which will promote choice? Something as apparently straightforward as allowing patients a choice of where they sit in the day room, or whether they eat their meals at the bedside or at a table in the ward can make a real difference to how the patients feel about themselves and their relationships with the nurses. Then gradually move on to consider areas of care which involve other groups and longer term discussion.

c. Reactions will differ. The accountability issue is important here. To offer choices and encourage independence will bring with it greater risks of accidents. If an elderly patient is allowed to sit in the day room when he wishes, there is a risk that he will fall over when no nurse is present. Is this an acceptable risk — to him, to you, and to the other staff who may be called upon to explain? Think out the possible objections in advance. Present a reasoned case for a specific change. It may help to introduce a new idea as a pilot project for a trial period. Usually it is a new attitude on trial, as much as a new behaviour.

d. Evaluation is never as neat as it seems in research reports. You will need varied sources of information. Are the nurses actually doing what was agreed — on your shift, on the other shift, on nights? How are the patients reacting? Criticism is hard to elicit, so take it seriously when it is given. Do the other professionals understand what you are doing and why? How does it affect them?

Conclusion

The way to produce change is through specific and well-prepared initiatives which are appropriate to your own clinical area. The key to working in partnership lies in changing attitudes; those of the nurses, those of the other professionals, and those of the patients themselves. Some nurses will argue that the idea of an equal partnership with patients is unrealistic. Certainly there will always be some patients who are unable or unwilling to be involved in their own nursing care. But the experience of community nurses is that many patients expect to be treated as equal partners, and this facilitates good nursing. Why should it be any different in hospital? Next time you hear a nurse saying, ''I'd like to nurse like that, but I don't have the time'', ask her how she will feel when it is her turn to be the patient.

Bibliography

Open University (1984). A Systematic Approach to Nursing Care. OU, Milton Keynes.
Chapter 4 has a good introductory section on the idea of partnership.
Bok, S. (1978). Lying. The Harvester Press, Sussex.
Excellent discussion of how to move from principles to practice in dealing with the complex ethical issues involved in allowing patients freedom to make choices.
Sanford, J. (1987). Making meals a pleasure. *Nursing Times* 83, 7, 31-2.
Some practical ideas on how to offer choice and begin to make changes.